MW01284052

STAY 40

without diet or exercise

Dr. Richard Lippman
Nominated for the Nobel Prize in Medicine

Outskirts Press, Inc.
Denver, Colorado

The opinions expressed in this manuscript are solely the opinions of the author and do not represent the opinions or thoughts of the publisher. The author has represented and warranted full ownership and/or legal right to publish all the materials in this book.

Stay 40
Without Diet or Exercise
All Rights Reserved.
Copyright © 2009 Dr. Richard Lippman
V4.0 R2.0 Third Printing

Cover Photo © 2009 JupiterImages Corporation. All rights reserved - used with permission.

This book may not be reproduced, transmitted, or stored in whole or in part by any means, including graphic, electronic, or mechanical without the express written consent of the publisher except in the case of brief quotations embodied in critical articles and reviews.

Outskirts Press, Inc.
http://www.outskirtspress.com

ISBN: 978-1-4327-2927-1

Library of Congress Control Number: 2008933715

Outskirts Press and the "OP" logo are trademarks belonging to Outskirts Press, Inc.

PRINTED IN THE UNITED STATES OF AMERICA

This book is dedicated to my children, grandchildren,
and M. Agneta Nilsson, RN

Acknowledgements

I humbly appreciate the knowledge and help bestowed upon me from esteemed doctors Ward Dean, Thiery Hertoghe, Jonathan V. Wright, Shannon Chang-Eaton, Clif Arrington, Ambjörn Ågren, Mathius Uhlen, Russell Laudon, Michael Brein, Jason Ako, and Garry F. Gordon. Also special thanks to my medical editor, Ward Dean, MD, and my literary editors John Nelson and Brian Fobi, PhD. I am also very grateful for the exceptional advice from America's foremost progesterone expert Michael E. Platt, MD, Europe's foremost endocrinologist Thiery Hertoghe, MD, and Britain's foremost pharmacist, Phil Micans. Lastly, I am indebted to the encouragement of Professor Denham Harman, MD, PhD, who inspired me to investigate the aging process some thirty years ago.

Disclaimer

The information in this book is based upon the research and professional experiences of the author. It is not intended as a substitute for consulting with your physician or other health care provider. Any attempt to diagnose and treat an illness should be done under the direction of a health care professional.

The publisher does not advocate the use of any particular health care protocol, but believes the information in this book should be available to the public as provided by the First Amendment. The publisher and author are not responsible for any adverse effects or consequences resulting from the use of any suggestions, preparations, or procedures discussed in this book.

Any decision made in relation to purchasing goods and /or services as a result of information obtained from the publication is your sole responsibility. The only warranty that we can give regarding the accuracy of the information is to state that all reasonable endeavors are made to remove inaccurate information from the publication to the best of our ability.

We will not be liable to any customer or member of the public for any information supplied in this publication. The publication is, provided on an "as is" basis and we do not make any representations or warranties if such information subsequently proves to be inaccurate or out of date. We cannot be held liable for any consequental loss resulting from the information we provide.

Should the reader have any questions concerning the appropriateness of any procedure or preparation mentioned, the author and publisher strongly suggest consulting a professional health care advisor, especially those knowledgeable in anti-aging medicine.

Foreword #1
By Dr. Ward Dean

I met Dr. Richard Lippman, author of *Stay 40 without diet or exercise*, at a *Gordon Research Conference on Aging* in 1982. Gordon Conferences are prestigious events involving specific scientific issues, and attended by many of the world's leading researchers in each field. I felt fortunate to have been accepted for attendance, and found myself surrounded by many of the most well-known and highly respected scientists in the gerontological (study of aging) scientific community, including such as doctors Roy Walford, Denham Harman, Johan Bjorksten, and many others.

One night I found myself sitting next to a young professor of biochemistry and cell biology from Sweden named Dr. Richard Lippman. We found that we had a number of similar interests. Both of us had great interest in the biological processes of aging, and we wanted to do something about it. During the 1980s most gerontologists approached aging as an intellectual exercise with little thought to practical application of their research findings. If anything, they seemed to be obsessed with producing long-lived cells, yeast, fungi, worms, rats, or mice with little apparent thought to practical application to human aging.

I recognized Dr. Lippman's name from a research paper that he had recently published, and at first thought that he was just another brilliant scientist engaged in an intellectual academic pursuit. However, I soon appreciated that Dr. Lippman was different. He consumed almost as many supplements and potential anti-aging drugs as I did. Although he applied himself to the research of aging on a fundamental cellular level, he also approached it with a practical eye towards extending human lifespan.

Since our first encounter over twenty five years ago, I met Dr. Lippman several times a year, usually at various aging-related scientific conferences. Over the years, I have encouraged him to write a book on the human potential of his anti-aging research, especially after his nomination for the Nobel Prize in Medicine.

Most of the popular anti-aging books available today have a problem. Their authors' main qualifications have often been reading someone else's anti-aging book. They have little or no experience themselves in conducting research or its application to humans.

Not so with Dr. Lippman or *Stay 40 without diet or exercise*. Dr. Lippman was a distinguished former professor of cell biology and biochemistry from the University of Uppsala in Sweden. He has performed basic research and authored a number of papers on free-radical chemistry and medicine in a search for an optimum combination of powerful antioxidants to retard the aging process and extend the healthy maximum human lifespan. More than just another "lab man", Dr. Lippman applied the knowledge gained from his research to himself, his associates, and his patients. All of his brilliant work led to a nomination for the Nobel Prize in Medicine for anti-aging research.

At last in *Stay 40 without diet or exercise,* he has organized the results of over a quarter century of research and clinical experience into a highly readable, entertaining, and insightful book from which all readers may find a number of valuable recommendations. These can be easily and economically applied to the betterment of their health, and the delay, and often even the reversal of their own bodily aging processes.

Ward Dean, M.D.

Foreword #2
By Dr. Garry F. Gordon

Dr. Richard Lippman has achieved many scientific breakthroughs during the past three decades. He invented the solar collector in Sweden in the early 1970s. He created the nicotine patch in the early 1980's, which has saved countless lives. He received the *first* American patent for nutrients he discovered that slow the human aging process. He was nominated for a Nobel Prize in Medicine in the late 1990's for his body of research on anti-aging. All of these achievements Dr. Lippman carried out with great energy and foresight, often in the face of skepticism from the scientific world.

But the most important of Dr. Lippman's gifts to us may be this book on how to extend human life. He has spent years -- decades -- aggressively tackling the aging process. What would you give to be free from the premature ravages of time? Imagine if you could extend your life to 100 years and beyond, and have decades more vital years.

Personally, I have known and respected Dr. Lippman and his revolutionary work since 1986. I met him many times at American Academy of Anti-Aging Medicine (A4M) meetings, which are attended by the world's leading scientists in anti-aging medicine. He amazed me with his encyclopedic knowledge of all areas of the field: chelation, hormones, antioxidants, free radicals, nutrition, and anti-glycation. Scientists recognize him worldwide for his proven and driven experimental genius as a researcher in all six areas. His dedication has made his work so important, not only for its achievements, but for what it dares to do. For example, Dr.

Lippman's 1987 patent entitled "Method for Retarding Aging" is the *only* American patent ever granted with claims for retarding human aging. This is an ingenious achievement, since, as a matter of principle, the US Patent Office never grants patents for perpetual motion machines and fountain of youth elixirs. Everyone in their first year of law school studies these "never granted" rules. Dr. Lippman breaks the mold and partially changes that hard and fast rule.

This book reflects his on-going passion to help people challenge the obstacles to a long, productive life. *Stay 40 without diet or exercise* opens exciting new doors that will enhance not only the quality of your life, but promises to add healthy future years to it. Dr. Lippman focuses all his scientific powers on the age-old question of why we age. You have met people who do not look their age, who appear much younger, or even older, than their true years. They have a secret: those who look younger really *are* biologically younger. They will live longer and healthier lives. Dr. Lippman's book teaches the reader how to recognize the signs of aging, and provides invaluable strategies and tools to conquer or reverse many of the most daunting road-blocks to long life.

He reveals how to manage the aging process and how to restore your body to youthful levels – all without plastic surgery. The methods described within will add years to your life and life to your years. Welcome to the brave new world of anti-aging therapy!

Garry F. Gordon, MD, DO

Contents

Dedication and Acknowledgements

Forewords by Drs. Dean and Gordon: Ward Dean, M.D., age 65, is a graduate of West Point and a decorated American military hero (Granada, 1983). Garry Gordon, M.D., D.O., age 73, is the father of chelation therapy since 1984. Both esteemed doctors have nearly thirty years experience treating the problems associated with aging.

Introduction to Dr. Lippman and his research

<u>**Section One**</u>**: The Science of Aging**

Section Two: Your Step-by-Step Plan to Staying Young

Section Three: Personal Finance, Pop Food Culture, & Health Promises of the New Millenium

Section Four: Appendix

An Introduction to Dr. Lippman and his new research

It was love at first sight.

The first time I saw Professor Denham Harman's research I was floored. I was amazed. He had managed to double the mean lifespan of lab mice by using *special* antioxidants. Other researchers had only extended lifespan by extreme diets and fasting.

Professor Harman had stepped out into the unknown, and I wished to join him. But how could I ride his coattails? I felt like The Time Traveler since no one else had any practical remedies for slowing aging. He did. I began to study chemistry, physics, and medicine since the esteemed Professor Harman demonstrated expertise in all three – not crazy diets and fasting. I needed to experiment like him, and perhaps clues to the aging process would reveal themselves.

Allow me to introduce myself. My name is Dr. Lippman, but my friends call me "Dick" or "Dr. Dick." For the last thirty-five years I have dedicated myself and my research to learning how to slow the aging process and provide more quality years to everyday people. Unlike my competitors, I have actually done anti-aging experiments and published in peer-reviewed gerontology (study of aging) journals since 1980, and like Professor Harman, my research has little to do with the pop culture remedies of diet, fasting, and heavy aerobics. Instead, my research has everything to do with understanding the aging process at the *cellular level*.

For many years, I lived in Sweden and attended leading institutions of learning. I studied chemistry and physics at the Swedish equivalent of MIT, namely The Royal Institute of Technology. Later, I studied medicine and did medical research at The Department of Medical Cell Biology, University of Uppsala, Sweden. I chose the career path of a scientist, and I studied the aging process with the best tools available to chemists, physicists, and medical researchers.

As in the case of Professor Harman, I have educated myself like a Renaissance man in these three disciplines and others; my remedies remain the most advanced and comprehensive you have ever heard. European and American scientists have told me many times that my research is light years ahead of the competition. During the last 30 years, my multi-disciplinary approach has allowed me and close colleagues to make the kind of breakthroughs in anti-aging research that others *only* write about.

These new breakthroughs have revealed that aging can be slowed, prevented, or even partly reversed. I have combined the best available methods to advance my knowledge of why and how we grow old. Unlike my competitors, I have used a hands-on approach and actually done the experiments. In contrast, most of my competitors have sat in their comfortable armchairs and used "Google" for obtaining their information since they often lack expertise outside of *general* medicine, diet, fasting, exercise, and nutrition. As a result, my book presents a multi-therapeutic approach where I explain at least 35 new and unique remedies for slowing aging and treating related health issues. You do not need to feel lousy and take handfuls of prescription drugs during your senior years. My regimen will make you happy. Hormones and other remedies will make you happy. Believe me.

Some of my remedies contributed to several inventions, awards, and accolades bestowed upon me during past decades. For example, I invented the nicotine patch in 1984 which I sold on national television. Secondly, I was awarded a US patent in 1987 for my anti-aging research – *the only US patent ever granted with claims for slowing the human aging process.* Thirdly, because of my innovative body of research, in 1996 I was nominated for the Nobel Prize in Medicine.

I invite you to open your eyes to some of the scientific wonders of the 21st century – wonders that can help you to slow, and occasionally even reverse, some aspects of aging. In beginning chapters I start with the simplest strategies that anyone can follow on a budget of less than 50 dollars a month. Then, I advance to more complex therapies that may cost more than 500 dollars a month. These latter strategies require testing and help of a knowledgeable anti-aging physician.

My strategies address the biggest concerns Americans have about growing older. According to *USA Today*, the number one fear was "slowing down", followed closely by unease regarding "overall health", and followed lastly by becoming a "family burden." I write for the layman, and therefore, scientists reading this book should forgive my abbreviated technical explanations. I try to write as simply as possible, but some scientific details may be difficult for the average reader. For all readers in a hurry, I summarize each chapter's recommendations at the end of every chapter for immediate implementation. For scientists, I detail clinical double-blind studies from prominent medical journals in the appendix.

If you sincerely want to avoid the ravages of aging, I offer you the most effective, comprehensive, *multi-therapeutic* approach possible, and my advice does not include dieting, surgery, handfuls of prescription drugs, or frequenting 24-hour sweat palaces. These methods I leave to the pop culture. My advice describes recommendations based upon my patent entitled *Method for Retarding Aging*. The following chapters reveal my new and remarkable remedies I offer to those who desire a change in their *rate of aging*.

A difficult problem exists in understanding aging at the cellular level. Physicians do not understand chemistry, and chemists do not understand medicine, and neither group understands much about free-radical physics. Each group is a specialty unto itself. Using my expertise, this book bridges the gaps between medicine, chemistry, and free-radical physics. It presents a multitude of methods that slow the rate of aging and the deterioration of our brains and bodies. It aims at extending the productive years of life, not the senile years. Life is meant to be a grand adventure, and by extending the productive years we can apply life's hard-earned wisdom to important pursuits. We should live life to its fullest in our later years and not end up vegetating with bingo, playing shuffleboard, and watching TV. We should remain participants and not voyeurs of life. Believe me.

For those of us NOT willing to go quietly into the night, I present in layman's language the best that cutting-edge anti-aging technology has to offer, namely 35 new remedies from my 30 years of research. My remedies will make you feel happy – reinstate your quality of life. You can avoid antidepressant drugs and feeling like crap until you pass away at age 90 or 100. Die healthy and have your brain at the end.

Believe it.

Medical information is doubling every four or five years with the likelihood that all *major* diseases may become curable in the year 2026. If we can only hold out to that significant year with the latest in anti-aging therapy and freedom from diseases, we may live long into the 21st century in good health. I am aspiring to do so, and I invite all other baby boomers with foresight and a willingness to change to join me in my quest.

Dr. Richard Lippman
Stockholm, Sweden
June, 2008

Section 1

The Science of Aging

Chapter 1
Understanding the Aging Process

Everyone wants to stay young. Everyone wants to live forever. Though these truths seem self-evident, every day most people engage in activities like smoking and eating high-sugar diets that shorten their lives. I have studied the aging process for over 30 years, and I now know that making changes can improve your chances of living a longer and more energetic life. These changes have nothing to do with the vanities of make-up or plastic surgery, but everything to do with the underlying causes of aging that take place at the *cellular level*.

Consider this: When doctors cure all major diseases in coming decades, the average lifespan will have only increased by *twelve years*. In other words, we will still be saddled with the same age-old problems of senility, wrinkling skin, loss of sex drive, and deteriorating but disease-free bodies. Our metabolisms will slow down, we will become less creative, more negative, flabbier, and scared of living and starting new projects. However, we can slow, or even reverse, these aging symptoms by understanding our cells' biochemical reactions and malfunctions that occur during aging. This understanding provides us with effective *remedies*.

Aging triggers profound changes throughout the body. At the *cellular level*, inadequate gene repairs lead to loss of cell reproduction and function, and eventually to death. Aging should be examined at the cellular level *first*, because changes there affect individual organs which, in turn, affect our entire body. One convincing theory explains our cells' reliance on oxygen metabolism, or how oxygen converts sugar to energy within every cell. This process creates **extremely poisonous chemicals called free radicals** that are exceptionally toxic to all. Indeed, the tragic aftermaths of Hiroshima, Nagasaki, and Chernobyl attest to the incredibly poisonous nature of free radicals – the strongest toxins on our planet.

Cell Death: Why We Age
Our hearts and brains decrease in size and lose function daily.
We call these changes aging.

Cell death is not in itself a bad thing. Every day millions of cells die and become replaced anew on the skin, scalp, mouth, throat, stomach, and intestine. However, cell death is negative in cells that do not reproduce and renew themselves. These cells are called *post-mitotic*, and one finds them only in the brain, heart and central nervous system. When thousands of these cells die or lose function daily, they are lost forever. Subsequently, our hearts and brains decrease in size and lose function daily. We call these changes *aging*. Fortunately, we have many brain functions and nerve transmission lines duplicated many times over so that we are unaffected by cell losses until our bodies reach a *critical age*. For example, imagine a young green tomato left out in the hot sun. First, it matures by turning red and shiny. Second, at a critical age it becomes dehydrated and its red skin wrinkles and loses its luster. Finally, it shrivels up completely into a dull, dark deflated sack good only for stewing. This critical age depends largely upon our genetic hand-of-cards dealt at birth. Our ancestors, especially on our mother's side, decide our reserves of these critical post-mitotic cells, and in turn, the future functioning of our hearts, brains, and other organs.

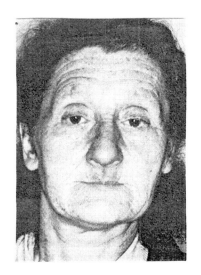 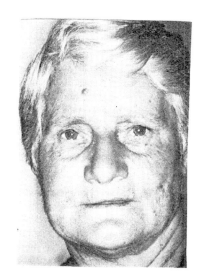

Figure 1. In comparing different people and how "old" they look, one may find an enormous difference between biological and chronological age. For example, the woman on the left is 45 years old who has aged much more rapidly than the 75 year old woman on the right.

Why We Die
Free radicals remain the likely culprits responsible for aging since they are the most poisonous substances in living organisms.

From the preceding description, aging may then be defined as gradual losses of *critical* cells in essential organs. When the loss becomes too great in a particular organ, it dies; in turn, without a transplanted organ, *we* die.

Alternatively, a vital organ may become weakened through *nutritional and hormonal deficiencies.* These two factors are the support troops in the battle of cell loss and death. Without these support troops, cells cannot function and they fade away and die. Two clear examples are deficiencies of Vitamins B12, D3, and testosterone in both men and women. B12 and D3 are critical for highly functioning brain cells; so when other people lose their ability

5

to absorb it through their intestines, brain function suffers and the brain shrinks.

Secondly, both men and women lose most of their testosterone production and other hormones from age 35 to 60. This loss promotes loss of libido, rough skin, and arterial vascular disease, especially in remote arteries in the legs responsible for our ability to walk. Thus, B12, D3, and testosterone critically support our mind, body, skin, and well being, and without their help we become impaired. We call this impairment aging.

The Essentials between Life and Death
Many illnesses associated with aging such as Parkinson's show loss of mitochondrial function, which means a loss of energy and cell death.

One may ask a very basic question regarding life and longevity: What is the essential difference between life and death? The answer seems surprisingly simple: energy. Every living organism uses energy. A dead organism has no energy. Energy originates from factories called the *mitochondria* housed in *every* cell of the body. The most physically active part of the body is the heart, and heart cells fill over one third their volumes with mitochondria. The heart also uses *Perkinje* cells as communicators that transmit pulses from the brain's *cerebellum* to the heart muscle. When these vital cells lose energy and mitochondrial function, a pacemaker must replace them or we die.

In the case of brain cells, similar energy losses occur. In these cells many illnesses associated with aging such as Parkinson's show loss of mitochondrial function, which means a loss of energy and cell death.

An intriguing question arises. If mitochondria are so essential to energy and life, what can we do to protect and even enhance their function? Since 1978 I have studied this problem, and I will explain my new research in coming chapters.

6

Our Biological "Clock"
Like the "Terminator," free radicals and their byproducts cause continual relentless damages to our tissues during many decades of aging.

From all corners of the globe, all animals and humans retain an extremely uniform rate of aging and dying. This fact suggests that one and only one biological "clock" determines aging. Look at it this way: If more than one "clock" controlled our aging, our rate of aging and dying would not be uniform. In other words, we would not have average lifespans of about 74 for men and 77 for women, or as written in the Bible, "three score and ten" (70) years. My unique research suggests that such incredible uniformity of lifespan between biblical and modern times must mean that only one "clock" works relentlessly and steadily ravaging our bodies until we wear out and expire. The most likely candidates are free radicals for continual relentless damages to our tissues during many decades. In our bodies, free radicals remain the most likely culprits responsible for aging due to their extremely poisonous nature and unstoppable 24/7 production.

For example, brief exposure to nuclear radiation generates free radicals and causes devastating cell damage and cell death (*necrosis*). A second example: try pouring hydrogen peroxide on your skin. Hydrogen peroxide is a byproduct of free radicals, and you will notice that upon contact with it your skin will temporarily become sickly white and *necrotic.* A third example is seen in older people who engage in very heavy aerobic exercise *without taking efficient free-radical scavengers – not vitamins.* Their muscles improve greatly, but their hair turns white and their DNA is damaged due to free radicals running amuck. All of these adverse changes are clear signs of biological aging.

Like the *"Terminator,"* free radicals and their byproducts do not stop. They cause continual relentless damages to our tissues during many decades of aging, and consequently, this biological "clock" determines our deterioration and eventual demise.

Anti-Aging Medicine Rescues Us from Orthodoxy
If our hormones become low and a flood of free radicals rages in our bodies, then we become susceptible to the diseases of aging and we rapidly age.

Anti-aging medicine seeks to rescue us from the relentless damages that our bodies have incurred after many decades of living. Through proactive steps known to anti-aging doctors, you can slow down, or even reverse, some of the processes of aging. Unfortunately, many of these tools remain unfamiliar to doctors of mainstream orthodox medicine since they are not taught in medical schools.

Indeed, in many ways the orthodox medical establishment remains philosophically unequipped to embrace the new paradigm of anti-aging medicine. It only encourages reducing risk factors by, for example, losing weight, fasting, stopping smoking, heavy exercising, and eating a Spartan diet. Also, most doctors practice palliative or "bed-pan medicine" meaning that they help the elderly become more physically and psychologically comfortable with aging and deterioration – a noble humanitarian pursuit, but an approach that limits more and healthier years.

On the other hand, anti-aging physicians have shown that these lifestyle changes solve *only part* of the aging problem – about 20%. The remaining 80% involves deficient hormones, tissue cross-linking, and inadequate defenses against free radicals.

Unfortunately, scientists have established that aging can only be marginally reversed by plastic *surgery* or *exercise*. Older people treated with facial aesthetic surgery will not result in their appearing dramatically younger. Plastic surgeons admit to achieving stellar results in less than 20% of their patients. Instead, patients will only appear more refreshed, invigorated, and look better for their age. In regard to exercise, older people must train excessively like athletes and make dramatic lifestyle changes in order to achieve a more attractive and youthful body. Also, heavy exercise without efficient free-radical protection ages them internally and externally on their heads and faces. This is evidenced by the rapid whitening of their hair and deepening grooves on their cheeks. If you doubt this statement, please examine the head and body photos in the excellent book, *Body for Life* by Bill Phillips.

As implied above, loss of vital hormones causes even serious pathologies. For example, aging cuts thyroid hormone in half, but you can successfully replace this and other declining hormones, with, for example, thyroid, testosterone, progesterone, DHEA, and human growth hormone. Consider the fact that ninety- and one-hundred-year-olds often have sufficient levels of hormones throughout their long lives, while those who die decades younger have lower, and often inadequate, hormone levels. This is my new and unique research. Hormones are the rate-limiting step that deficiencies prevent most of us from living to at least our nineties. Consequently, these super seniors have high levels of hormones and healthy cells. For example, Okinawa women live longest on the planet with an average lifespan of 86 years. Blood levels of their hormones at age 100 revealed that their testosterone is more than double that of average 70 year old American women. Believe me, hormones, and free radicals are critical to understanding the aging process.

Numerous scientific publications document well a dynamic and obvious association between hormone deficiencies, toxic free radicals, and aging. Indeed, if our hormones become low and a flood of free radicals rages in our bodies, then we become susceptible to the diseases of aging and we rapidly age. To avoid this syndrome, knowledgeable anti-aging physicians treat the entire body with multiple anti-aging remedies. This is my special idea, and by "remedies" I do not mean treating the skin with expensive creams, Botox and collagen injections, and plastic surgery. Interestingly, *extra* vitamin supplements do not affect your *rate* of aging unless you face starvation in a third-world country. Also, I do not mean treating sleep disorders with drugs, and depression with antidepressants. Instead, I treat the underlying causes of aging and not just its symptoms.

So far I have described what free radicals and hormones do on the *cellular level*. Allow me to explain their effects at the *tissue level*. For example, women often have declining levels of the natural female hormone *estradiol*, especially after menopause. At the tissue level, thirty year old women have approximately 50 or 60 layers of tissue in the walls of their vaginas. Those tissues are healthy and well lubricated with a slightly acidic (pH) environment. On the other hand, women at age eighty have only about eight tissue layers

9

remaining. Those tissues have become dry and open to bacterial and yeast infections due to cell loss and increasing alkalinity (pH). Also, their external skin becomes very thin through loss of collagen. Both loss of collagen and shrinkage of vaginal layers can be prevented and partially reversed by restoring natural bio-identical hormones (BIH) such as *estradiol* combined with *progesterone.* I am not talking about patent drugs like medroxyprogesterone or expensive cosmetic creams and lotions. BIHs are hormones that Mother Nature produces naturally in both plants and animals. One may restore and reinstate them in the human body with the help of a knowledgeable physician. On the other hand, one should not substitute these natural gifts of nature with synthetic drugs produced by the pharmaceutical industry. These drugs will alleviate some hormonal problems, but often they will be accompanied by unwanted side effects since the human body recognizes them as alien. Natural estradiol reinstatement truly tightens and moisturizes the skin as Mother Nature intended, and even a little natural progesterone and testosterone helps too. Interestingly, the monthly cost of bio-identical hormones – not drugs – is typically less than what women spend monthly for cosmetic creams and lotions. Again, it is your choice. Believe the advertising of the cosmetic or drug industries or join the more informed anti-aging revolution.

You can solve these problems of cellular and tissue damages and aging through a more comprehensive and scientifically advanced approach. This approach has become possible today thanks to recent and sophisticated *measurements* of an individual's hormones, amino acids, free radicals, peroxides, and cross linking. For example, the recent development of special 24-hour urine tests allows measurement of no less than twenty-nine hormones and their metabolites. (*Note: A 24-hour urine test means collecting your total urine output during a 24-hour period, and then mailing in two small test tubes for analysis to a special lab.*) This comprehensive profile has become critical to understanding an individual's complete hormonal needs and means of correcting them. Thus, for those serious about anti-aging, I always prescribe special 24-hour urine tests. It is your choice.

In any case, the quickie approach with a simple blood test may be the best way to start on a limited budget paid by your health ;urance. Later on, one can further fine tune a comprehensive anti- ıg strategy with the more detailed 24-hour urine tests.

10

History and Popular Misconceptions About Aging
*Ask any orthodox physician about curing your aging symp[
and he or she will respond with an emphatic
"NO. We only treat disease."*

Until recent times, when it has become an obsession, the quest for eternal youth has usually been regarded with cynicism and even derision in Western culture. In the 16th century, Spanish explorer Juan Ponce De Leon haplessly searched for his fountain of youth in the swamps of Florida, but to no avail. In the 19th century, Oscar Wilde's *Picture of Dorian Gray* treated the preservation of youthful beauty as a wicked indulgence. In the early 1920s, surgeons grafted monkey glands onto the torsos of aged men in an attempt to replenish their hormones, but these experiments went largely unnoticed by the medical community. In the 1930s, Harvard scientists demonstrated that lab mice could double their lifespan if fed *only* on alternate days, findings that startled many. Then starting in the 1940s, Swiss doctors began injecting famous people, such as Winston Churchill, with live cells harvested from newborn lambs in an effort to regenerate declining organs. In the 1950s, the father of modern anti-aging medicine, Professor Denham Harman, proved that mean lifespan could be more than doubled by feeding lab mice *strong antioxidants* and not just Vitamins C and E. This breakthrough study initiated the most productive area of anti-aging research including my own unique findings.

In spite of productive advances, the general public remains largely uninformed about the steps they can take that will *really* make a difference. Or, we're exhorted to revere the "*joys of aging*" or to be contented with one's aging despite obvious evidence to the contrary confronting us daily in the mirror. This is nonsense.

Believe your own eyes while observing the people coming and going in public places such as beaches and airports. Sagging facial skin and jowl lines often distinguish those over 40 years old since Mother Nature wants to destroy our bodies. Melting faces represent clear symptoms of aging and at the cellular level indicate a lack of DHEA, Igf-1, and human growth hormone (HGH). One prominent expert told me that "beaches and airports have become museums for exhibiting hormonal deficiencies." Believe it.

Aging is clearly not a disease, but a natural process that begins in our mid twenties. Therefore, the well-meaning but orthodox medical community often cannot help patients with their aging symptoms, since they have been taught at medical school to address *only* diseases. Ask any orthodox physician about curing your aging symptoms, and he or she will respond with an emphatic "NO. We only treat disease."

Protecting Ourselves against Cell Loss and Aging
We can consume different nutrients that hinder cell breakdown, membrane damage, and consequent cell death

Nature has provided us with a wide variety of natural *lines of defense* against destruction of our membranes and consequent destruction of cells critical to our health and life.

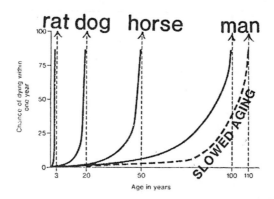

Figure 2. The chances of dying as a function of age in mice, dogs, horses and humankind.

In my own research I have found that the higher up on Darwin's scale of evolution, the more elaborate and compartmentalized are an organism's *lines of defense*. They consist of different enzymes and nutrients. These hinder cell breakdown, membrane damage, and consequent cell death. Scientists often call them hormones, strong antioxidants, membrane stabilizers, stem cells, and anti-cross linkers.

A More Rational Approach to Anti-Aging Medicine
"Men occasionally stumble over the truth, but most of them pick themselves up and hurry off as if nothing had happened." —
Winston Churchill

At present, an oceanic divide exists between the conventional medical approach to aging and those who specialize in anti-aging medicine. On the one shore, conventional medicine focuses upon healing the sick with the latest patented drugs. On the other shore, doctors knowledgeable in anti-aging medicine advocate slowing aging by replacement with nutrients and bio-identical hormones often already employed by Mother Nature. And that makes all the difference.

Understanding this difference has become the most urgent scientific challenge of our age. The tragedy of Americans slowly fading away into the dark scourge of old age has become unconscionable to 21st century anti-aging physicians. It is time to seek inspiration from the leaders of the anti-aging movement, starting with two-time Nobel Prize winner, Dr. Linus Pauling, the pioneer of modern anti-aging medicine and chemistry, Professor Denham Harman, and the foremost pioneer of practicing anti-aging medicine, Ward Dean, MD.

These and other pioneers (including myself) have researched and compiled an extensive library of clinical double-blind studies that support anti-aging remedies detailed in this book's appendix. These studies are based on more than seventy years of research beginning with the discovery of natural testosterone in 1934 and the first curing of glaucoma with adrenal extract in 1937. Most doctors are unaware of these studies unless they are current with hormone (endocrinology) and anti-aging research often detailed in America's leading medical journals such as NEJM and JAMA.

Anti-aging medicine is the real McCoy, and one should not associate it with some of the patent medicines and cosmetics touted endlessly in the media. Keep in mind that more than half of all clinically double-blinded drugs registered in the US between 1975 and 1994 had serious side effects. Indeed, according to the October 22 issue of *The Archives of Internal Medicine*, up to four times as many side effects have been discovered by independent researchers compared to claims made from drug-company paid researchers. Consequently, prescription drugs are the fourth leading cause of death in the US after heart disease, cancer, and stroke[1].

In fact, prescription drug related deaths are more common than highway accidents, breast cancer, or AIDs. By contrast, other modern industrial countries such as Sweden and France severely restrict drugs with significant side effects. It is high time to put aside outdated prejudices and accept significant advances from independent scientists and medical researchers as reported in America's leading medical journals.

Medical knowledge is doubling every five or six years, and the American Academy of Anti-Aging Medicine has predicted that all *major* diseases will become curable by 2026. This prediction is unnerving given the reluctance of orthodox medicine to examine and employ pragmatic advances reported in current medical journals. Our modern outlook appears radical to all those cemented in the conventional practices of the past.

In the following chapters, you will read about unique substances that my research has uncovered — and my special research methods for measuring and monitoring them — that can keep you healthy and happy until 100 years or older.

In summary, I am firmly convinced that the *three major causes* of the human aging process are:

(1) A deficiency of hormones
(2) Cross linking (glycation) of tissues
(3) Inadequate defenses against toxic free radicals.

You will also learn about the many other minor causes of human aging as we go along. Underlying these causes is the indisputable fact that *hormones* plunge after age 50 in everyone. Women especially become susceptible to heart disease and osteoporosis. Studies show that men gain visceral fat, lose muscle mass, and develop heart problems.

Double blind placebo-controlled studies demonstrate unequivocally that reinstatement of hormones to levels of younger people is essential for living healthier lives. For example, during the first century AD, wealthy and sexually dysfunctional Roman women applied to their genitals gladiator perspiration and oils that were rich in androgens. (According to a 2002 University of California at Berkeley study, the perspiration of athletes contained the hormone androstenediene that raised levels of cortisone in women who used it.) Then the Chinese in the eleventh century applied a similar hormonal residue obtained from the urine of young men and women. Only recently have Americans rediscovered and updated lost hormone replacement techniques from the ancient Romans and Chinese.

In addition to hormone replacement, the prophylactic use of STRONG free-radical scavengers and anti-cross linkers further inhibit the aging process. By employing the latest cutting-edge remedies presented in this book, you can defeat or at least delay many of the problems associated with aging.

I invite everyone to join me in my adventure to a healthier and happier life. Preventative anti-aging medicine is fast becoming a heroic medical art form whose radiant achievements hold a promise of renewed health and longevity.

Golden keys to longevity #1

- *The reader may avoid many aspects of aging and related diseases by applying anti-aging medicine. This new medical specialty encourages prevention of many age-related problems. The reader can achieve optimal health and longevity by balancing and reinstating hormones, preventing and reversing cross linking, and strengthening lines of defense against toxic free radicals as detailed in coming chapters.*

End Notes: [1] JAMA, Journal of the American Medical Association, Jason et. al., Vol. 279, April 15, 1998, pp. 1200-1205. Also JAMA, Bates, David, W., Vol. 279, April 15, 1998, pp. 1216-1217.

Chapter 2
Busting A Few Myths

Irrational Exuberance, Cherished Beliefs and Maddening Notions of the Crowd

People need myths. The contrived stories that we tell sooth a psychological need. Karl Marx once wrote that religion is the opium of the masses, but today many Americans turn not to God, but to other unfounded beliefs in order to assuage their fears during periods of rapid technological advances. Long before they invented science and engineering, people relied upon myths to sustain them and carry them through life. Fortunately, we have shrugged off some myths such as, "the sun revolves around the earth," and "Columbus was the first to discover America." While exposing myths can perhaps seem intimidating or even frightening, doing so can also open entire new worlds of possibility.

Are you ready to shrug off further misconceptions about aging and health care? Hold on to your seat while I debunk some myths armed with recent advances gleamed from prominent medical journals. I will right now only briefly touch upon remedies for aging because in later chapters I will flesh them out in greater detail.

Let us start with my Canadian buddy, John, and his all-too-common beliefs about his life and his aging.

Myths of Testosterone
Cardiovascular and genital health depends upon adequate amounts of testosterone.

One day I had a friendly meeting with my buddy John from Canada. We joked about sports and our dating experiences. He liked to kid me about my eccentric habits of not owning a television. I enjoyed teasing him about his Montreal hometown and the rabble-rousing habits of French Canadians who often threaten to secede from the dominion of Canada. Later during our conversation, I gently posed the subject of impotence in men as they grow older.

John flashed a mischievous smile. He claimed to have lots of testosterone (T), and he seemed unconcerned about impotence or erectile dysfunction (ED) as he grew older. He freely joked that his potency depended upon the beauty and charms of the woman in his presence. I became serious and pointed out that men lose two thirds to three fourths of their testosterone between the ages 35 and 60, and the consequences are dire. John again smiled ear to ear and intimated that he remained a macho man with lots of libido and passion for women. I injected that if he did lose T, his erections would become softer, and this condition would also indicate cardiovascular damage throughout his body.

During aging, men often experience large losses of T and some cardiovascular damage since the body loses T-producing *Leydig* cells. Cardiovascular and genital health critically relies upon adequate amounts of testosterone.

Adequate supplies of T also affect women. It is a myth that T is only a man's hormone. Older women especially need T replacement back to the levels of their twenties. Many senior women I know began to feel sexy again when supplementing with as little as 5 mg of T gel daily. T allows intimacy again for all post-menopausal women taking T, and their husbands sure enjoy a renewed sexual intimacy too. Interestingly, older women with facial hair have a significant advantage over women without since this condition often signifies adequate amounts of natural T that also protect women's arteries and heighten their libidos. In other words, the bearded lady at the circus has uniquely high levels of T and extra sex drive.

However, allow me to explain a word of caution regarding

women and T. Women only need *adequate* amounts of T, which is about one twentieth as much as men require. Women should not supplement above their normal T values since extreme doses of T may cause breast cancer. Instead of high dose T, women should balance their estrogen hormones and protect themselves from breast cancer with other hormones such as *progesterone* and *estriol*. Nature intended this natural course of action as explained in Chapter One.

Many men like John remain content with their myth of high libido supposedly determined by the charming lady at their side. Then they hit their 50's and 60's, and Mother Nature plays the dirty trick of putting a crimp in their sex lives. Subsequently, Big Pharma enters the picture touting in endless television commercials about the temporary benefits of the drugs, *Viagra®*, *Cialis®*, and *Levitra®*. These sex aids sound like three rock stars. I used to recommend them until I discovered the incredible potency of bio-identical T combined with the libido hormone *oxytocin*. Forget the myths and fantasies of Canadian John, and join the bio-identical hormone revolution. The 21st century has arrived and natural hormone replacement with T has become one of this century's many longevity miracles -- My Lippman Promise.

The Myth That Cosmetic Sprays and Creams Will Maintain Youthful Skin
Natural hormones keep your skin soft without expensive cosmetics.

The cosmetic industry perpetuates the biggest myth of all in terms of dollars spent: Namely, during aging women need daily treatment with creams and sprays for healthy, moist, youthful skin. Nothing could be further from the truth. The cheaper and natural way to youthful skin is for women to take all natural hormones such as *thyroid, testosterone, and estradiol.* 80% of aging women are thyroid hormone deficient. Many of these women truly need the estrogen, "estradiol" in the form of a daily applied gel. Many physicians also prescribe a little *estriol* and *progesterone* which complement and balance estradiol. *Estradiol will firm and tighten sagging skin within a few months use – all without plastic surgery or moisturizing creams.* Low dose testosterone in women (4 to 7 mg daily) will keep a woman's skin soft without an expensive moisturizing cream. Mother Nature intended women to avoid aging skin and loss of collagen with natural, bio-identical estradiol and testosterone creams. Believe me; estradiol, testosterone, and thyroid replacement works without need of cosmetics.

Some women have enough of these hormones generated naturally by their bodies throughout their entire lives. Sophia Loren is a prime example of a celebrity who has escaped many aspects of tissue aging due to an adequate and natural supply of hormones. Unfortunately, most women do not have Sophia's exceptional hormones, and they should reinstate their hormones to remain youthful with lots of collagen and thick, moist skin.

The Big Lie: If You're Older Than Age 45 and Feel Tired and Lethargic, Your Doctor Writes You a Prescription for an Antidepressant
Do not buy into this frightening myth. Beware of any product heavily touted with the words "medroxy" or "conjugated."

This incredible lie is perpetuated daily on thousands of Americans, especially women. Antidepressants will alleviate your symptoms of fatigue and lethargy -- namely prevent uptake of brain serotonin in order that more free serotonin is available for brain energy -- but a better solution exists. That better solution addresses the underlying cause of low serotonin, namely declining hormones during aging. Aging people lose many of their hormones, and they begin to feel like crap. This "like-crap" feeling continues until the day they pass away unless bio-identical replacement therapy is employed by knowledgeable physicians. Unfortunately, uninformed medicos will prescribe *synthetic* (chemically altered) hormones such as *medroxyprogesterone* to alleviate symptoms such as hot flashes and depression. This is a mistake, and it betrays a lack of knowledge of bio-identical hormone replacement therapy.

Many physicians do not understand the difference between natural remedies versus synthetic drugs. Indeed, **medroxy**progesterone (Provera®) causes cancer according to the Women's Health Initiative Report in 2002; while natural progesterone showed no signs of any malignancy. In fact, natural progesterone is the live-long estradiol since they balance each other and work synei together to promote optimal female health. This important V health report has been often misinterpreted by the press and ₚₒp culture. Further clarification has been sorely needed. Finally, a 2007 French study of 10,000 women (Breast Cancer Research & Treatment; Vol. 1, pp. 125-134) revealed that women who used estradiol combined with the synthetic drug, Progestin, had almost double the incidence of breast cancer than women who used the natural hormones, estradiol and progesterone.

Interestingly, another synthetic hormone, namely *medroxy-testosterone*, caused cancer in men during the 1950's, and it was pulled off the market for its horrendous side effects. "**Medroxy**" and "**methyl**" synthetic hormones are the origin of the myth that natural testosterone causes cancer; while in reality, only synthetic hormones are to blame. Apparently, "medroxy" and other synthetic hormones have a long history of injury to the American public extending back more than half a century, but those adverse histories have been quickly forgotten or misunderstood. Do not buy into this frightening myth. Beware of any product heavily touted with the words "medroxy" or "conjugated" in their patient information sheets. Your life or that of your loved one may be at risk.

The Myth That Natural Hormones Will Harm You
All physicians should feel an ethical duty to become better informed.

Bio-identical hormones (BIH) are completely natural since they are extracted from Mexican yams by the pharmaceutical giant, Pharmacia-Upjohn. Then they are made into creams, gels, and capsules by specialty pharmacists called "compounding pharmacists." In contrast to synthetic drugs, BIHs remain harmless to us since they are identical to hormones already existing in our bodies, and they have been successfully employed for millions of years by all plants and animals on our planet.

Despite what you may have read in the press or heard from uninformed doctors, natural bio-identical hormones are safe, while synthetic (chemically altered) versions of hormones may be unsafe. In the appendix, I list prominent double-blind clinical studies that support my claims. The same is true of strong antioxidants and anti-cross linkers. These substances and BIHs will promote a healthier and happier life; other remedies – especially patented synthetic drugs – will shorten your life especially if used long term.

Physicians should become knowledgeable about advancements in anti-aging medicine and advise their patients accordingly. Failure to use anti-aging remedies – especially estrogen in women, and testosterone and Armour thyroid in both men and women – will result in loss of hair, nails, skin, strength, muscles, energy, well-being, and protection from some types of cancer. All physicians should feel an ethical duty to become better informed of advances in the medical journals.

The Myth that Extreme Diet, Nutrition, and Heavy Exercise Will Slow Your Rate of Aging
Fasting every other day will damage you.

Many popular books promote the idea that extreme diet, nutrition, and heavy exercise will slow aging. This statement contradicts many scientific studies. For example, residents of Honolulu, Hawaii, live twelve years longer on average than people in New York City and ten years longer than people in Washington, D.C. Obviously, people of Honolulu do not exercise more than their North American counterparts; nor do they diet more, consume more vitamins, or follow special nutritional fads.

Clearly other factors of aging or slowed aging account for this ten- to twelve-year discrepancy. This book will outline the whys and wherefores of this discrepancy as well as how we can truly slow our rate of aging. As proposed by several popular books, my methods will not require you to starve yourself by fasting every other day. In 1935, Cornell University scientists discovered this restrictive starvation diet when lab mice were fed on alternate days only, and their lifespan increased by about fifty percent. Such is not the case in humans, and I know this for a fact since several prominent anti-aging physicians have died or suffered shortened lifespans and health

22

problems by fasting every other day. I have nothing against occasional fasting, but fasting every other day will damage you. Trust me.

The Myth That All Antioxidants Enhance Health and Longevity
Weak antioxidants such as Vitamins C and E do not increase lifespan.

Another common myth promoted by advertising since the early '90s is the one concerning antioxidants. According to media hype, every third product in health food stores is a *good/better/best antioxidant.* This modern myth has persisted despite attempts by me and my fellow scientists to dispel this absurdity.

I understand the wrongness of this hype. Long before advertising became involved; I spent many years developing new and unique medical instruments for *measuring* suspected antioxidants in living organisms. My first measuring method employed special chemical probes that targeted the insides of our cells where toxic free radicals are continually being generated. My second measuring method used near-infrared spectroscopy, which allowed measurement of fat peroxides in humans. By careful measurement and analysis of free radicals and fat peroxides, I obtained *exacting* knowledge of strong and weak antioxidants and their effects upon health and lifespan.

My new findings allowed me to formulate *powerful* antioxidant or free-radical scavenger mixtures, which were duly registered with two medical authorities, namely the Swedish and Italian FDAs.

Furthermore, I discovered that weak antioxidants such as Vitamins C and E do not increase lifespan. This information flies in the face of marketing ploys from vitamin manufacturers claiming that vitamins extend lifespan. Believe me, they do not. Adequate amounts of Vitamins C and E remain essential for health, but extra supplements may adversely affect your longevity. As a result of the confusion concerning antioxidants, I use only the alternative phrase, "*free-radical scavengers*" throughout this book.

Marketing hype uses repetition to seduce us. If one tells the same lie often enough, most people become true believers – a key principal of the German philosopher Friedrich Nietzsche.

Cholesterol Myths That Put Your Life on the Line
Did you know that half of all heart-attack sufferers had "normal" cholesterol values?

The news media has incredible powers of persuasion, and those powers have been directed NARROWLY to promoting cholesterol-reducing *statin* drugs. This myopic focus results in the widespread belief that heart disease can be remedied by the statins. Wrong. Did you know that half of all heart-attack sufferers had "normal" cholesterol values? *Heart problems are often not caused by high cholesterol but low T3 thyroid hormone.* Other critical factors of cardiovascular disease completely ignored by the media and even some doctors are:

- Low T3 thyroid
- Chronic inflammation.
- Excessive blood coagulability.
- Elevated homocysteine.
- Lack of Vitamin D3.
- Deficiencies of hormones: melatonin, testosterone, estrogens, cortisol, DHEA, progesterone, insulin, EPO, human growth hormone, etc.

Middle age and older people risk their lives if they remain untested for the above factors. Testing is simple, but proper diagnosis may be difficult for physicians not trained in anti-aging medicine. Your doctor may order common blood tests which determine C-reactive protein, fibrinogen, homocysteine, thyroid, Vitamin D3, and lipoprotein-particle-size.

The news media's narrow focus on the statins has resulted in a near epidemic of drug side effects including *fibromyalgia* or muscle weakness. Many prominent cardiologists are aware of these facts, and consequently, they only prescribe statins to middle-aged men with advanced cardiovascular disease — despite incredible marketing pressures from some drug companies. Unless you fit this restricted category, find a qualified cardiologist or anti-aging physician who will test you for C-reactive protein and other factors listed above.

In the meantime, if you care about your health and longevity, please consume daily a healthy diet dominated by fresh fish, low carbs, daily exercise, 2 to 3 grams daily of the spice *turmeric*, a minimum of 150 mg of *CoQ10*, and 250 mg/d of the *chelator*, EDTA. These are my new and special research recommendations.

Interestingly, the best substitute for statin drugs are a minimum of 2 grams daily of non-flush Vitamin B3 or niacin. The Harvard Medical School has researched and endorsed this remedy, since niacin has the additional benefit of increasing the good cholesterol, HDL unlike the statins. Statin drug sales remain a multi-billion dollar industry despite cheaper and safer alternatives. Strangely, we ignored the research of a leading medical school in favor of relentless hype from the drug industry. Very strange. I will explore this subject in greater detail later.

The Myth That *Heavy* Aerobic Exercise Benefits Longevity
When our body becomes overwhelmed by free radicals, damage occurs especially to the vital non-reproducing cells of the heart, brain, and central nervous system.

In the course of my research, I discovered other interesting phenomena that dramatically affect longevity. I determined that *heavy* aerobic exercise damages our bodies. By "heavy exercise" I mean excessive expansion and contraction of the chest causing over eight times normal the amount of oxygen consumed. For example, a two-mile high-speed run around the park will cause this excess. Unfortunately, this eight-fold oxygen increase in intake generates huge quantities of oxygen free radicals in our cells that overwhelm our bodies' lines of defense. When defenses become overwhelmed, damage occurs especially to our vital non-reproducing cells of the head, heart, brain, and central nervous system. Especially in older people, hair whitens and faces appear to age rapidly during the course of less than one year of heavy aerobics as evidenced by Bill Phillips excellent book, *Body for Life*, 2008.

Of course everyone requires daily exercise for a normal healthy life. However, excessive "eight-fold" exercise generates free radicals and puts us in harm's way which may result in stroke, heart attacks, white hair, and long-term damage to our vital organs. The worst result is *"sudden death syndrome"* or sudden heart attacks suffered by seemingly healthy joggers. Believe me, sudden death syndrome has nothing to do with elevated cholesterol and everything to do with the eight-fold increased generation of oxygen free radicals.

Free radicals are Death's Protégées. Invoking them with eight-fold heavy exercise causes cellular damages – micro-insults to our critical non-reproducing cells of the heart, brain, and central nervous system. In our youth, stem cells, juvenile cells, and hormones replenish and rebuilt our bodies, but less so during aging. Do not invoke eight-fold free-radical cascades. Avoid the myths of the 24-hour sweat palaces and instead exercise moderately along with consuming EFFICIENT free-radical scavengers 24/7. These reduce your chances of sudden death syndrome and long-term organ deterioration.

Myths of Some Omega-3 Fatty Acids
Big Pharma still uses ethyl-mercury as a preservative in vaccines routinely injected into even frail seniors.

One finds omega-3 fatty acids in flax seeds and fish. They should be healthy but often fall short of touted benefits due to pesticides in flax seeds and mercury in fish. Also, flax seeds contain the inflammatory fatty acid, *omega-6*. Therefore, I strongly advocate consuming fish everyday and eliminating mercury. We can easily eliminate mercury and other heavy metals by *"chelating"* or removing them with such substances as *EDTA* and *DMSA*. The web site at www.vrp.com further explains and sells these important nutrients. If we refuse to clean fish of mercury, we will endure some long-term nerve damage. Indeed, some seniors have become so full of mercury-damaged nerves that their hands tremble when they lift light objects. Other seniors have difficulty reacting quickly to dangerous traffic situations. A tragedy.

And the worst of it occurs during the fall season in the US. Even frail seniors are routinely injected with flu vaccines loaded with an *ethyl-mercury* preservative. This same preservative caused birth defects in the Middle East fifty years ago. I remember studying this

tragedy in my first year at medical school. Such uses of mer
unconscionable and strictly forbidden in European countries. w...
will the US wake up to poisons like mercury?

Do not become a mercury junky. I remove mercury routinely
from my brain and other tissues with an excellent chelator called
DMSA. Please consume at least 250 mg before or after any fish meal
or before any flu shot — or receive your flu shots in Europe like I do.

Pesticides such as *PCBs* have also become a problem. I have
extracted pesticides from flax seeds and other grains and seeds by
chemical removal methods. For example, in the coffee industry,
caffeine is routinely removed by extraction with *chloroform*.
Unfortunately, trace residues of chloroform remain in decaf coffee,
and we ingest these residues when we drink decaf. Indeed, some
friends of mine such as my Canadian buddy John, accept low-level
quantities of pesticides since they become stored in body fat, and
thus rendered harmless. This fat storage eliminates them from the
immediate chemistry in our cells. Rather than accept pesticides in my
body fat, I prefer fish where I eliminate mercury up front with
chelation. Your choice.

In addition, I choose to add nutritional support to my brain with
mercury-free fish oils instead of oils from junk burgers. This is my
newest research conclusion. Junk burgers damage health as revealed
by several recent documentaries involving fast-food restaurants. I
expect my brain to function well into my nineties and beyond if I
recharge it daily with fresh fish oils and not oils from junk burgers.
Your choice.

Myths of Depression in Seniors
*Do not believe the myth that depression in seniors
is only solved by treating with antidepressants.*

Recently, I read an article about a large clinical study concerning
depression and suicide among American seniors. This very large and
well documented study concluded that suicide and depression are six
times as likely in those over 65 versus those younger than 65. Also,
four-fifths of all suicides were men over the age of 65.

The study concluded that physicians and therapists should better diagnose and treat those over 65 with anti-depressants. I agree that this course of action is a worthy pursuit for treating **symptoms** of depression and suicide, but it ignores the underlying **causes**. The underlying causes are lack of testosterone (T) and a general imbalance of other hormones. In men, T falls from about 1100 to1400 pg/ml serum (blood) at age 19 to about 250 to 350 after age 60. Senior men become especially depressed and suicidal, especially when their serum T falls below a threshold value of 288 ng/dl (see references in Chapter 5 table). This threshold value also places senior men at extreme risk for Alzheimer's disease, arterial stiffness, Type II diabetes, and an approximate 8% thickening of their carotid arteries according to the latest research during the last four years (see table references in Chapter 5). Because of T's importance in regulating mood and happiness, when T levels sharply decline in aging men, they can become depressed and contemplate or commit suicide. The stereotype of the grumpy old man is not so far off. Indeed, as men age, they often become grumpy, and their wives are quick to exclaim, "He is not the man I married!" Declining testosterone is the culprit, and reinstatement with bio-identical T is the solution. On the other hand, senior women seem to cope better when their T declines since they can fall back upon their female hormones, the estrogens.

Do not believe the myth that depression in the elderly is only solved by treating symptoms with antidepressants. Bio-identical hormone reinstatement works best, especially in the case of men replacing their testosterone.

Myths of Binge Eating
A long and healthy life rests upon consumption of low-calorie and low-sugar balanced diets Americans previously ate.

Many people harbor the illusion that every day they are eating normal and healthy food portions. In fact, studies have shown that the average American eats 3,900 calories daily, but they believe they're eating only 1,800 calories. People unconsciously binge eat despite evidence to the contrary. Time to bust this myth.

Indeed, as a consequence, two thirds of Americans are overweight, and one out of five Americans is headed for Type 2 diabetes – a horrendous national tragedy that remains unacknowledged by many. People enjoy the myth of binge eating high-sugar diets in spite of obvious negative consequences. One day I remember discussing the problem with ordinary people assembled in a coffee bar.

A retired lady said that she had worked many years as a waitress beginning in the '60s. She inspired me to question her about the dietary habits of Americans back then. I asked her to remember the type of food she served when she first started waitressing. She recalled that food portions were smaller and contained less sugar. Indeed, as a boy in the mid-50s I remember visiting a restaurant with my father, and we were served only a few *thin* pancakes or waffles in an order called a "short stack". She said that this order was common back then, and food habits had indeed changed dramatically in the '70s when everyone started ordering those awful thick Belgian waffles and pancakes with gooey, undercooked centers. Yuck.

Something was amiss. The food industry had run amuck. Such seemingly innocent changes had encouraged many Americans to consume heavier diets to the detriment of their health and longevity. And the worst of it was increased sugar consumption and risk of diabetes.

She and I reminisced about other dramatic changes in the way Americans eat. We could remember eating at McDonalds in the late '50s when the soda sizes were only 5 and 9 ounces instead of super-sizing with today's 12, 16, and 32 ounces of sugar water. Clearly, Americans had deluded themselves into consuming heavy foods rich in sugar, and few seemed to care or reflect upon those crazy changes. Time to bust this myth and declare that a long and healthy life rests upon consumption of low-calorie and low-sugar *balanced* diets Americans previously ate.

If you doubt me, please try screening movies from 1930 to 1960 where the actors appeared very thin relative to modern ones. Remember the "zoot suits" from the early '40s that accented v-shaped builds? During the first half of the 20th century, both men and women appeared more "v-shaped" than today revealing narrow waists and correspondingly wide shoulders. Another good example is the viewing of beachgoer photos from past decades.

We ought to discard the modern habit of heavy eating with high gar intake if we hope to live long well into the 21st century. We do not need these large portions of sugary foods. With determination and concern for my own health and longevity, I have eliminated these foods from my diet, and so can you. And there are millions of people in neighboring industrial countries that do manage to stay thin and healthy by avoiding sugar and large food portions. One really only needs large food portions if one is a farm hand or construction worker.

Recently a diabetic patient phoned me from another state, and asked me what I recommended as a long-term remedy for his sugar problem. Since he lived in a city with a large Asian population, I suggested that he eat only Asian food. Asians who keep to their traditional cuisine and avoid North American food will remain lean and out of harm's way from diabetes. The Asians I treat who are overweight usually eat North American food and often abandon their Asian foods. Consuming Asian food is the no brainer method for avoiding Type 2 diabetes.

Myths of Cures for Sleep Problems during Aging
Solving these problems is accomplished by employing Mother Nature's most natural of all remedies.

Many, many times I have heard that no cures exist for the common malady of teeth grinding and clenching of teeth, especially during sleep. These sleep problems are common during aging. In the short term, some sufferers have found relief with the anti-anxiety medications like Clonazepam®. However, this only addresses temporary relief from symptoms. The underlying cause is simply high levels of serotonin and cortisol – these cause anxiety as well as a host of other sleep disorders such as sleeplessness.

Do not buy into this myth. Solving these problems is accomplished by employing Mother Nature's most natural of all remedies: the bio-identical hormone *progesterone*. Bio-identical progesterone -and not horse-urine drugs (Provera®) - naturally calms the mind and body and maintains hormonal balance. Progesterone is also the natural life-long partner of estrogens such as estradiol. For women, I recommend about 100 mg daily dose of *bio-identical* progesterone cream ordered from licensed compounding pharmacist as listed in the resource section of this book. For men, I recommend about 40 mg daily since high doses may adversely affect their erections.

Bio-identical progesterone cream really works for long term relief of teeth grinding and other sleep problems associated with aging. One hour before bedtime, try rubbing it into the jaw with at least ten forceful strokes. Further sleep enhancement benefits become available when 0.5 mg if the sleep hormone *melatonin* and 50 mg 5-hydroxy tryptophan added to the progesterone cream. A third method common in Europe employs chamomile cream rubbed vigorously into the jaw. These work.

The Myth That Orthodox Physicians Can Correct Your Aging
Forget the myth that any ordinary physician can
solve your aging problems.

As explained in the first chapter, orthodox medical practitioners are not equipped philosophically or educationally to address your aging because it is a natural process and not a disease. Understandably, physicians have nobly dedicated their lives to curing disease but not slowing a natural process like aging. They might further educate themselves in the new medical specialty of anti-aging medicine according to the following example.

Recently at an age management convention, I met a very warm and charming conventional cardiologist, Tom, age 63. He explained his personal need for understanding anti-aging medicine since both he and his daughter needed help. He asked me to explain how he might become educated in this new medical specialty. I recited a partial list of nutrients and drugs used *prophylactically* for all those over the age of 50. He pressed me further, and I explained the necessary doses for age management of Baby Boomers. He stated that as an orthodox cardiologist, he was unfamiliar with many of the non-drug nutrients used. I replied that learning the use of anti-aging drugs combined with nutraceuticals (non-prescription drugs) takes time and effort, and I suggested several educational courses for

31

physicians. Of special importance is special testing, such as 24-hour urine tests which measure and monitor no less than 29 hormones and their metabolites. Furthermore, I encouraged him to begin an anti-aging practice first upon himself with known medical tests and prescription drugs, and when his knowledge increased, he could stepwise add nutraceuticals to his approach.

He thanked me for my timely advice, and promised to keep in email contact with me. Indeed, according to Harvard educated anti-aging expert, Jonathan V. Wright, MD, at least a thousand anti-aging educated physicians are needed in the coming years to address the needs of the Baby Boomers. Forget the myth that any ordinary physician can solve your aging problems. Education is the key, and in coming years I will do my best to fulfill that need.

In summary, ordinary physicians cannot help you with your problems associated with aging unless they are committed to years of additional study in the specialty of anti-aging medicine. Anti-aging medicine is a very complex subject, much like nuclear physics and rocket science.

The Myth of Accurate Medical News
*Few seem to realize that this is a form of advertising,
and not journalism.*

Politicians use the phrase "spin-doctoring" which describes the act of putting the most biased, slanted and sometimes even dishonest interpretation of political news and events. The same happens in the arena of medical news. The news media announces "wonder drugs" which later turn out to have exaggerated or insignificant benefits. Indeed, in 2004 the FDA approved 480 new drugs, but only 30 of them were actually new and unique while the remaining 450 were more or less copies of older drugs.

We do not expect that medical news would be an outright fabrication, but such is often the case. TV news stations are hungry for stories about medical breakthroughs. They receive film clips from their parent network, news service, or a public relations company providing sound bites containing "medical news." They seldom question the original source of the "news" which is often a drug company. Drug companies are only too happy to comply with slickly written and produced film clips touting the latest benefits of a drug while understating its side effects. For example, Wyeth-Averst promoted their combination weight lost drug fen-phen® by hiring people to ghost write stories about the miracle of fen-phen dieting without explaining significant side effects which were well known at the time. My sister took fen-phen and fortunately quit before suffering the long term consequences of heart damage. Unfortunately, hundreds more died, and many more were badly hurt.

Public relations companies churn out an abundance of misleading spin-doctored medical news, and TV stations swallow it willingly without checking out its authenticity. Though you would imagine that educated and dedicated doctors would resist these crass attempts at persuasion, this so-called news does have an impact on how they treat their patients. Sadly, few people recognize this as a form of advertising, and not news. The public's only weapon is an internet search of the government's Medline which will often reveal many side effects of any given drug if known – assuming that the researchers in question have not juggled statistics or engineered research protocols to produce a desired outcome. Alternatively, one may ask a trusted medical doctor if the "medical news" seems credible. In any case, a wait-and-see attitude is best. Avoid spin-doctored news for a healthier and happier future.

The Myths of Treating Symptoms
and Not the Underlying Disease
These physicians spend time actually listening to their patients and conducting extensive testing.

Once we reach forty years old, Mother Nature attacks our bodies with a vengeance. Our metabolism slows down, our skin gets wrinkled and flabby, muscle mass decreases, and fat increases. We become more negative and less likely to start new and creative projects. Heart attacks and strokes kill half of us, and cancer kills one out of six. Despite popular myths to the contrary, Americans are 42nd in the world in longevity and 37th in health care. We grow older much faster since many have multiple hormone imbalances and

33

cascades of free radicals revealed as *clusters of symptoms.* If we take these clusters of symptoms to most conventional doctors, they will offer us a Motrin and send us home! Motrin is great for relieving temporary pain, but it does not address our underlying problems of raging free radicals and multiple hormone imbalances. For this therapy, we need to find physicians trained in preventative medicine and especially those knowledgeable in anti-aging medicine.

If you do not believe this, consider all those patients today taking multiple medications with horrendous side effects. Statistically, more than half of all prescription drugs newly registered from 1975 to 1994 have serious side effects, except for the year 1989. Indeed, 1989 was the one and only year in which more than half of all newly registered drugs did not have serious side effects. Hurray. Consider all the women of today with rampant problems of miscarriages, breast cancer, fibroids, and coronary artery disease. This would become unnecessary if we treat the underlying causes of these problems and not just the symptoms. Unfortunately, if one only treats symptoms, damages occur, and sometimes irreversibly so.

Into this wasteland of limited treatments and knowledge has walked a new type of physician who treats underlying causes of diseases and not just symptoms. These physicians spend time actually listening to their patients and conducting extensive testing such as the aforementioned blood and urine tests. Your typical HMO medico will refuse this service since they operate under tight budgetary restrictions from their masters, the health insurance companies. Unfortunately, these companies demand "managed care," which means tight testing budgets and limited patient visits. As a result, quick treatment of symptoms with the latest patented nostrum has priority in their world of managed health care.

The physicians practicing "real" medicine are those who take time for their patients, test them extensively, and address their underlying problems and not only their symptoms. They will honor The Hippocratic Oath where physicians swear to, "treat the sick to the best of one's ability." Often they will be prescribing natural bio-identical hormones and only occasionally synthetic drugs. They will ribe such natural remedies as *iodine* tablets, which studies ested are the reason that Japanese women have lower rates ncer than American women.

In summary, the following facts are uncontroversial. During the last 50 years, studies have shown that hormones plunge dramatically in men and women, especially after menopause and andropause (male menopause). Muscle mass decreases and osteoporosis and fat increase dramatically. Numerous clinical studies demonstrate that this condition leads to heart disease. However, many experts have clung to their cherished beliefs and ignored landmark double-blinded studies that reveal the tremendous benefits of natural hormone reinstatement.

Myths of Prostate, Breast, and Uterine Cancers
JAMA concluded that treatment was based upon the services provided by the doctor rather than the superiority of the treatment.

Prostate, breast, and uterine cancers are growing in the populations of Western countries, especially prostate cancer. Often treatment depends upon which medical specialist a patient asks. For example, in 2000 the Journal of the American Medical Association (JAMA) carried an article comparing the treatments of urologists with radiation oncologists in men with prostate cancer. 92% of the urologists recommended removal of the prostate gland, while 72% of the radiation oncologists recommended radiation. *JAMA concluded that treatment was based upon the services provided by the doctor rather than the superiority of the treatment.* Also, neither group advised nutritional or hormonal treatment. Apparently, little thought is ever given to the underlying causes of these cancers. If the causes were identified, then more appropriate remedies could be employed. This same thinking especially applies to hypothyroidism and cancers of the breast and uterus. I have many stories to tell regarding these afflictions.

Not only is conventional medical treatment overly impacted by the specialty of the treating physician, but the profession as a whole remains fixated on maintaining the unproven fact that testosterone causes cancer. The 31 references on testosterone in the appendix attest to the true fact that testosterone does not cause cancer. Trust me. If high testosterone levels cause prostate and other cancers, why do not male teenagers get prostate cancer? Apparently, the myths and prejudices of the past century still dominate, and some people are having a difficult time adjusting to *current clinical double-blind evidence.*

The truth is that as men age, they lose about three-fourths of their testosterone (T) while their estrogens remain about the same. This creates an estrogen dominance known to increase the risk of prostate cancer and the swelling of prostates. Also, when T declines during aging, men increase their fat cells, especially around the stomach. These fat cells produce even more estrogens, and thus, estrogen fuel is added to the fire – the fire of *estrogen dominance.*

Estrogen dominance stimulates prostate cell growth in men as well as breast and uterus cell growth in women. Still another source of rising estrogens is from an overabundance of false or pseudo-estrogens from plastic residues and pesticides such as PCBs and dioxins. We need to remedy these rises since *estrogen dominance is the only known cause of uterine cancer.*

The male equivalent of the uterus is the prostate gland. Indeed, both glands developed from the same embryonic cells, and thus, it is not surprising that both remain under the same hormonal influences – ditto breast cells. All contain the same cancer-causing gene (oncogene Bcl-2) as well as the cancer-protecting gene, p53. Today effective methods exist that will discourage the cancer causing gene and encourage the cancer protecting gene.

Prominent medical journals have revealed these facts within the last decade, and thus, they remain unknown to many. In future, it should become common to *block* the cancer causing gene and promote the cancer protecting gene. This has become a significant goal of anti-aging therapy. Specifically, I encourage the blocking of the estrogen, *estradiol,* in everyone estrogen dominant. There are many types of estradiol blocks available such as bio-identical progesterone, estriol, DIM, Indole-3-Carbinol, Arimindex®, and especially 2-methoxyestradiol (2ME2). For example, 70% of breast cancers are driven by aromatase activity which can be inhibited by DIM, Indole-3-Carbinol, and Arimidex. Recently, according to the Mayo Clinic, 2ME2 "has shown promise in treating sarcoma, lung, and brain cancers, demonstrates that the drug may also be effective in treating breast cancer, in particular the spread of breast cancer" (*Science Daily* 11/04/07). It is also effective in treating leukemia, *osteosarcoma, chondrosarcoma,* and prostate cancers e have spread to the bone (see appendix references).

These blocks help to rebalance all hormones so that estrogen dominance subsides. Furthermore, other hormones such as thyroid, melatonin and testosterone are often added to achieve balance. Also, proper nutritional support becomes essential for all rebalanced hormones since a good diet remains the cornerstone of highly functioning hormones. These steps should help to prevent many cancers in both men and women.

Let us get a handle on aging for living better and longer lives. We need to focus on the causes of illness rather than the symptoms. We should be relying on prevention and not "rescue medicine." Instead of waiting for the diseases of aging to strike, become proactive, preventative, and optimize your hormones and other nutrients. Remember that health is not merely the absence of disease or symptoms, so we must take proactive steps to insure health and longevity and slow the processes of an aging future. You must take responsibility for your own health and longevity by educating yourself and taking action on a daily basis.

Golden keys to longevity #2

Despite the myths of modern life:

- *Avoid high-sugar diets and farm-hand portions.*
- *Avoid statin drugs.*
- *Avoid heavy aerobic exercise.*
- *Consume efficient free-radical scavengers such as l-acetyl cysteine.*
- *Use hormone replacement therapy, especially OPTIMAL amounts of bio-identical testosterone and other hormones that are balanced with one another.*
- *Support your brain and body with fresh fish and fish oils and please eliminate mercury. Find physicians who truly listen to their patients, test extensively, and prescribe medications that solve underlying problems and not only symptoms.*

Chapter 3
Prevent Cross Linking and Slow Your Aging!

The Discovery of Cross Linking and Aluminum in the Brain
Cross-linking explains why skin wrinkles and arteries harden at a rate of about 7% per decade.

The origin of my meeting Dr. Johan Björksten is cast in obscurity, while his discovery of cross linking remains a myth to some and a revelation to many – an epiphany to all those who love advances in science.

I do remember having many engaging conversations with him over bowls of borsch since he favored Russian restaurants in his hometown of Helsinki, Finnland. He was a reserved man who spoke sparingly in English, but became quite verbose when speaking Swedish, his native tongue. We had many long discussions in eloquent Swedish. During one meeting on a grey cloudy day with the pavement wet from an early-morning rain, my six-year-old son and I stepped off a rickety trolley and walked the cobblestone streets of Helsinki. The feeling of Russian/Stalinist dominance over this fair Scandinavian city disturbed me.

We met Dr. Björksten at a Russian bistro commonplace throughout Finland. Standing in the doorway, very tall, gaunt and blond, the famous Finnish scientist greeted my son André and me with a warm smile and sparkling blue eyes. He described with passion his latest research on aluminum's role in the deadly business of Alzheimer's, a disease rendering many a capable brain into a blackened, jellied mass of plaques and tangles. Ionized aluminum somehow enters the brains of the innocent and wreaks havoc by *cross-linking* vital neurons essential for thinking and movement. I became so engrossed in the pearls of wisdom falling from his lips that I was oblivious to everyone around me. What the great scientist said became magic to my young scientific mind. Eventually, he paused and glanced strangely to my right side. I followed his eyes to discover that André had fallen asleep with his handsome head face down in a bowl of Russian borsch.

These fateful meetings encouraged me to study the role of the metal aluminum and why it causes accumulations of oxidized fats found in vegtable oils, meats, and humans. In addition, I studied other metals and their roles in aging and oxidized fats. This inspired my research and encouraged me to understand why skin wrinkles and why brains become senile with age. Before I met him, my research focused on the brain's storage of *plaques* during aging and especially with Alzheimer's. Plaques are composed of rancid fats which accumulate from the oxidation of fats such as *LDL* (*low density lipoprotein*), commonly referred to as the "bad cholesterol." The esteemed Dr. Björksten encouraged my understanding of brain, artery, and skin chemistry. I revered this man. Dr. Björksten doggedly devoted 50 years of his life to uncovering the mysteries of *cross-linking*. With his help, I linked together the sciences of chemistry and medicine to better understand human aging. He also inspired an awareness of the *cross-linking* or combining of proteins with sugars in the entire body, whether human or animal. Cross-linking explains why:

- leather hardens and loses elasticity during the tanning process.
- paint hardens and loses elasticity during the drying process.
- the skin hardens and becomes inelastic from decades of sun exposure.

- the lens of the eyes harden and lose elasticity from decades of sun exposure.
- skin wrinkles and arteries harden at a rate of about 7% per decade. Thus, the maximum potential lifespan is about 140 years when arteries become 100% hardened.
- hardened and cross-linked tissues such as blood vessels are increasingly likely to rupture as in the case of stroke.
- essential proteins and molecules form tangles and become biologically inert during aging.
- the cells become increasingly burdened with malfunctioning and inert molecules which cannot be removed, and they hinder intercellular transport. This sets the stage for some adult-onset diseases of aging.

High Blood Sugar Causes further Damages
Subsequent high blood-sugar level results in many of aging's infirmities, namely degeneration of the eyes, damage to blood vessels, and shortening of life span.

Forty years ago, Dr. Björksten's discoveries became important, and they encourage my research, much to the betterment of society. Such are the rewards of science. During the 70's, he discovered that aluminum molecules dissolved from common aluminum *cookware* were implicated in Alzheimer's disease. From there, he elegantly deduced the adverse roles of glucose, sugars, and proteins in the formation of permanent *cross links* in the brain and body. From this groundbreaking work, other scientists discovered that the nutrient *aminoguanidine* prevented cross linking and other aging effects.

These scientists identified aminoguanidine in the slowing of diabetes. Type 2 diabetes—involving a sugar called glucose— is an accelerator of the aging process. High blood sugar results in many of the infirmities of aging, namely degeneration of the eyes, damage to blood vessels, and shortening of life span. Please skip over the following scientific box if uninterested in chemistry.

41

The Scientific Explanation of Cross Linking (Glycation)

Our body is built structurally with proteins. Some proteins with free *amine* groups become reversibly bound to glucose and other sugars. These compounds can easily return to their original state of separated amines and sugars. However, during normal aging or in the case of accelerated aging (diabetes), they oxidize to form permanent *amide* compounds. At the molecular level, these amide compounds are what we call cross linking, and they become visibly apparent during aging and accelerated aging (diabetes) in the form of wrinkled skin, hardening of the lens of your eyes, hardening of your arteries, and impairment of your heart and kidneys.

Fortunately, these adverse effects partially reverse themselves by *aminoguanidine* or its synthetic cousin *Metformin®*. These are known in the scientific literature to alleviate or prevent senile cataracts, heart and arterial thickening, kidney failure, skin wrinkling, thinning bones, osteoarthritis, and a host of other degenerations which we often label as simply aging. But conventional medicine often ignores these striking results.

Cross linking remains high on my list of the primary causes of human aging – make no mistake.

Beefing Up Insulin Receptors and Preventing Diabetes
Personally, I would like to know if my insulin receptors have lost sensitivity, so I could do something about it.

Diabetes has become the scourge of our country, and one fifth of all Americans are destined to acquire it. In New York City, the victims will rise to one out of three. This is a coming epidemic more widespread than AIDS. We become diabetic by eating heavy sugar diets which damages our bodies, especially our insulin receptors. Everyone over the age of thirty should be tested for this potential damage with a simple blood test called HB-A1C. Without this test, many people over thirty became sub-clinically diabetic, and they often remain unaware of it until a medical emergency strikes. This is much like the aging process: We remain largely unconcerned about aging until one of the diseases of aging strike us down.

Fortunately, subclinical diabetes lends itself to effective treatment. However if left untreated, this gradual and insidious process results in the slow deterioration of our life-supporting arteries. This causes their hardening and consequent rise in our blood pressure. If allowed to continue unchecked, this process escalates into full-blown diabetes which may result in blindness and leg amputation. Believe me.

Allow me to insert a brief case history from the files of my friend and colleague Dr. Ward Dean MD, one of the country's leading anti-aging physicians. For more than two decades, he has treated patients for their aging symptoms with many of the nutrients recommended in this book. Also, he has written several books himself on brain enhancement. He and I have worked hand in hand for decades advancing the science of anti-aging medicine.

His patient, Mr. Madson and two of his siblings developed Type 2 diabetes before the age of fifty. Both had neurological diseases called *neuropathy* and *retinopathy*, respectively. Mr. M questioned the efficacy of goat's rue for diabetics which Mr. M wished to recommend to his siblings. Dr. Dean pioneered the research on the benefits of goat's rue, a natural herbal substance with fewer side-effects than Metformin, a common prescription drug for diabetes. Specifically, Mr. M asked Dr. Dean what scientific evidence he had that goat rue or aminoguanidine really worked.

Dr. Dean responded:

"That's a good question. Admittedly the data on goat rue is pretty sparse and quite old. The anti-diabetic drug Metformin employs the activity of aminoguanidine which gives the herb, goat's rue or French lilac (galega oficinalis) its anti-diabetic properties. I have not seen any recent studies with goat's rue; however many clinical studies conducted recently with aminoguanidine and its synthetic derivative, Metformin show positive results. Using goat's rue, I have only anecdotal evidence from my patients that attest to its efficacy."

Mr. M decided to try goat's rue and later blood tests showed lowered blood sugar. The highlights of Dr. Dean's research on goat's rue can be found at www.thehealthierlife.co.uk. Please skip over the following in the scientific box if uninterested in science:

Scientific Explanation of the Benefits of Aminoguanidine

Aminoguanidine is known to prevent age-related heart enlargement in animals. It reduced 30% below normal the heart's membrane surface, and furthermore, the collagen content of the heart's arterial walls increased 24% to 30% above normal.

During the last twenty-five years, studies at the University of Milan have shown that aminoguanidine reduces the ability of low-density lipoprotein or LDL to bind itself to blood vessel walls. This action prevents blood platelets from coagulating and forming dangerous clots. Diabetic clinical trials with humans have highlighted its ability to prevent oxidative changes in LDL and inhibit the formation of atherosclerotic plaques.

Third, aminoguanidine has the ability to improve the health of patients whose blood vessels are constricted by arteriosclerosis. At the University of Milan, doctors treated eleven patients with peripheral vascular disease with aminoguanidine. Their blood vessels were so clogged that they could not walk for more than 500 meters. But after treatment, their blood flow improved an average of 30%, and their ability to exercise improved 50 to 105%. *Because cross-linking can double or triple, many people rightly view diabetes as a form of accelerated aging.*

Lastly, aminoguanidine can significantly reduce *albuminuria* as evidenced by proteins found in the urine as a result of kidney disease. It also delays the onset of end-stage renal disease and improves the cholesterol profiles of diabetic patients.

Preventing Aging Means Preventing *Glycation*
We become stiff in our muscles, skin, and arteries as we age, and this cross linking can be remedied using several anti-glycating agents.

Alan, 53, worried about the cross linking of his skin and the hardening of his arteries as he grew older. He had read conflicting reports about the dosage of carnosine needed to correct his *glycation,* or cross linking. Some doctors recommended 50mg two to three times daily, while others insisted that he take 500mg, an amount which gave him headaches. He wondered if he would benefit from the lower dosage.

I explained that Dr. Mario Kyriasis, a noted expert on carnosine, recommended 50 to 200mg daily. At this dosage, patients lowered their free radicals and made general health improvements. On the other hand, children with *autism* seemed to benefit from doses of 800mg daily. Indeed, life-extension folks often employ one gram, or 1,000mg, daily. High dosages in lab animals attest to carnosine's low toxicity, and the above dosages seem safe. While I usually recommended higher doses for maximum benefit, I told Alex that his body knew best: the headaches could indicate that his cross-linking remained limited, and a lower dose should deliver the necessary benefits.

From this study and many others scientists now realized that *glycation* means unwanted cross linking or binding of sugars with proteins. Also, glycation affixes glucose to membranes, hemoglobin, and other structures where it can severely impair their functions. Scientists can easily reproduce this process in a test tube or the human body since its chemistry has been well studied for over a hundred years. A common test uses hemoglobin A1C. This process explains why we become stiff in our muscles, skin, and arteries during aging. Thanks to Russian and British scientists, glycation can be remedied using several anti-glycating agents. One special type, called carnosine, is effective, but aminoguanidine works better according to my unique research and that of the eminent British pharmacist Phil Micans. See Figure One.

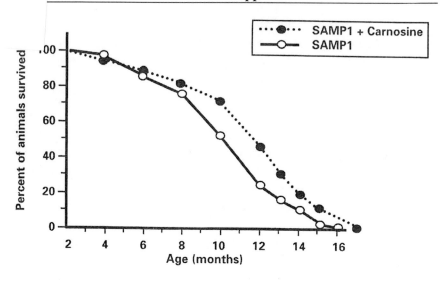

Figure One. Carnosine extends the lifespan of SAMP1 mice by several months. (Yuneva, et. Al. 1999)

According to Dr. Micans, aminoguanidine should be used in any anti-aging regimen in early stages; while carnosine and pyridoxamine work better in late-stage therapy. Any serious anti-aging program would employ all three nutrients in total dosages of less than 700 mg daily, spread throughout the day and taken on an empty stomach (my new research).

We concluded that aminoguanidine has the potential to slow damage to the body's proteins with advancing age, and more so in the case of full-blown diabetes. Furthermore, it protects the proteins of the body, especially the kidney and lens of the eyes proteins, and those of the skin, namely *collagen, elastin,* and *hyaluronic acid.* Some of these effects can be measured by the instruments that I invented and described in more detail in coming chapters. Allow me to interject another case study here, one of many from our files.

A fifty-eight-year-old volunteer in normal health consumed daily 300mg *carnosine* and 15mg *resveratrol* and soon appeared to have the circulatory system of a younger man. After abstinence from these nutrients, this volunteer's cross-linking parameters (blood viscosity, biological age, etc.) began to return to a normal fifty-eight-year-old's level. Other double-blind tests indicated that aminoguanidine showed even greater benefits. Personally, I consume resveratrol, carnosine, and aminoguanidine 24/7, and you should too. After several months, you should notice improvements in balance, blood pressure and blood sedimentation rate.

These nutrients are truly valuable to anyone serious about slowing their aging. During an 18 month period I used these three anti-cross linkers, and my blood pressure improved from 118 over 80 to 118 over 60 (millimeters of mercury). In other words, anti-cross linkers improved my blood pressure from the normal values of a very healthy 60 year old to those of a typical teenager.

Further Food for Thought
Thanks to the interaction of many scientists, prevention and reversal of cross-linking is fast becoming essential to any serious anti-aging program.

The science of anti-aging medicine employs a very human process that for decades has required the cooperation and inspiration of many researchers seeking new answers to age-old problems of aging. Such research has uncovered special nutrients that slow, prevent, and even reverse the effects of protein and sugar cross-linking. These special nutrients are having a major impact upon preventive medicine, especially in the treatment of sub-clinical diseases. Thanks to the interaction of many scientists, prevention and reversal of cross-linking is fast becoming essential to any serious anti-aging program.

I am *chronologically* sixty-three years old, but my body measures *biologically* several decades younger and remains disease-free. My blood pressure and sed rate are the same as teenagers, namely 118 over 60 and 3, respectively. My muscular strenght and balance are also very youthful: I can stand on one leg blind-folded for several minutes while the norm for 60 year olds is only an average of 10 seconds. Try it yourself.

I have managed to hinder and reverse cross-linking and glycation, and this has allowed me to physically engage myself like a youngster. I enjoy dancing, and my flexible body can dance and twist

... n to the one-foot limbo level above the dance floor. I enjoy playing jump rope with my grandchildren, and I manage to jump the rope 22 without faltering. To be clear, I am no athlete, nor have I had much interest in sports. My true passions encompass science, art, foreign language, and history—all rather sedentary activities. Hindering or reversing cross linking permits greater agility, and I invite you to join me. A healthier and more elastic future can be yours too.

Golden Keys to Longevity #3

- *The French consume lots of cheese and pasteries yet they are much thinner than Americans due to their consuming seventeen percent less sugar and engaging in more sexual activity. Low sugar consumption means less cross linking, more agility, and better health, especially if combined with special anti-cross linkers.*

Recommendations

- For anti-aging only, start with ultra-low dose *aminoguanidine* or *Metformin*, 75 - 150 mg daily. For experienced anti-agers: use min. 250 mg daily *l-carnosine* plus 15 mg/d *resveratrol*.
- Consume *only* unsweetened fruit juices such as grapefruit or pomegranate. Cut back on all sources of sugar which includes both sucrose (table sugar) and fructose (sugar in fruit), and the worst of all: high fructose corn syrup used laviously in most coffee houses and fast-food restaurants. Substitute these for *xylitol* sugar, my favorite, available in small packets at vrp.com, or my sister's favorite, stevia.

Chapter 4
Is It Dangerous to Breathe?

Protect Yourself from Free Radicals:
The Strongest Poisons On The Planet

"The only reason I would take up jogging is to hear
heavy breathing again." Erma Bombeck, humorist

Daily Bombardment of Free Radicals Causes Damages
I became convinced of the efficacy of truly strong free-radical
scavengers to reverse long-term damages.

Did you know that your body suffers *daily* an average of 7,000 free-radical attacks? In the prominent medical journal *Nature*, recent research has found that free radicals are implicated in a growing number of ailments, especially atherosclerosis, inflammation, plaques, cancer, insulin resistance, Crohn's disease, ulcerative colitis, and Alzheimer's[1].

Our bodies burn pounds of oxygen daily which generates huge cascades of free radicals 24/7. These cascades hit your brain, arteries, organs, and genes, and they cause damage unless defended against by special *lines of defense*. These lines become increasingly complex as one moves up the evolutionary ladder from bacteria to mammals, and finally to humans. A Darwinian struggle has occurred over millions of years that progressively improved our vital *lines of defense* against free-radical damage. Through the process of natural selection, many species were eliminated in favor of those who evolved elaborate lines of defense against free radicals. Humans and other mammals that evolved increasing resistance to poisonous forms of oxygen were blessed with longer life spans and healthier brains. This is my unique research conclusion. Also, these developments increased our ability to acquire knowledge, develop tools, and form civilizations as we know them today. Our elaborate lines of defense acquired from our ancestors became our genetic inheritance. We can strengthen them and our brains by consuming truly *efficient* free-radical scavengers, not Vitamins C and E.

As mentioned in the Introduction, I did research for many years at the Department of Medical Cell Biology at the University of Uppsala in Sweden. I became interested in artery and cell damage through my collaboration with the pharmaceutical giant Pharmacia, long before they merged with Upjohn to become Pharmacia-Upjohn. Pharmacia had a very active program studying *ischemia*, which means narrowed blood vessels and decreased oxygen in the brain, arteries, and other tissues. They developed a technique for demonstrating clearly the role of free radicals in decreasing the flow of oxygenated blood. Without harming their lab hamsters, they would inject them with an innocuous dye and anesthetic. Then the thin skin of the hamsters' cheek pouches was gently laid over a light microscope. Through the lens of the microscope, one could observe in real time the blood flow through extremely fine blood vessels. During the second phase of this experiment, a solution of *superoxide anion radicals* was rapidly injected into these fine blood vessels. A camera recorded the gradual narrowing of these fine blood vessels due to free radical damage. Scientists call this ischemia (*narrowed blood vessels*), and it is critical to tissue health. Make no mistake.

During the experiment's third phase, a solution of strong free-radical scavengers such as l-glutathione was injected into these narrowed blood vessels, and the damage completely reversed itself. I became an "ischemia enthusiast" since this work clearly demonstrated the critical importance of free radicals in the proper functioning of our organs.

As a young scientist, these decisive experiments convinced me that free-radical scavengers were extremely important to the blood vessels. I became absolutely certain that truly strong free-radical scavengers reverse damages caused by ischemia (*narrowed blood vessels*). I was elated to have participated in these revolutionary discoveries. Pharmacia guided me on the right track in pursuing an area of study largely neglected by other researchers. This was a new and unique moment in my researching career. Bridging the sciences of organic chemistry, medicine, and free-radical physics allowed me to truly understand ischemia, and I became highly educated in all three disciplines. My research advanced to the betterment of mankind. The importance of free radicals to cell and organ health is priceless. Believe me.

My Case Study of Free Radical Damage
After a single EDTA bath, she doubled her time outdoors by removing metals that catalyzed free radicals and caused her skin to burn.

By the time Ms. Smith arrived at my weight loss program, she had fought a losing battle for years. She remained fat, and as the fat girl at school she was an outcast. Lately, she had become reclusive with her extra eighty pounds. A true American tragedy.

I solved her binge eating problems by putting her on my weight-loss patch called "*Slim Patch.*" I created this patch due to the strong response to my nicotine patch invention. I counseled her about the dietary changes, especially the need to add fresh fish to her diet. This balanced her sugar cravings and the extra fish raised her metabolism by about 20%. Changing to a healthier diet corrects many hormonal and other problems within 24 hours. With these problems resolved, she still had difficulties with *free radicals*. She loved sunbathing, but she would easily burn. I suggested that she try 250 mg daily of the free-radical scavenger, *l-glutathione*. Also, she should bath weekly in a warm tub containing two grams of *EDTA powder*. Also, EDTA is a chelator (remover) that bonds to the metals, copper, mercury, iron, and cadmium in her skin. After a single EDTA bath, she doubled her time outdoors by removing metals that catalyzed free radicals and caused her skin to burn. EDTA helps to eliminate inflammation and sunburn. This was my special research results. Decades of sun would have shriveled her skin like a dried prune – thus the down side of skin damage caused by sun-induced free radicals. This shriveling process is also accelerated by deficiencies of such hormones as HGH and testosterone.

Ms. S thanked me and allowed me to use her photos in my diet program. I had made her happy and protected her skin from free-radical damage. Surely the everyday problems of aging, weight control, and skin are complex and overlapping, and too often the medical community sends patients home with advice such as "eat less and stay out of the sun." Anti-aging physicians offer patients more than a string of worn-out phrases.

Famous Hollywood actresses have had their skin renewed – not by cosmetics and plastic surgery – but by the treatments advocated in this chapter.

Aging and Free-Radical Damage to Your Cells
Their huge reactivity makes them a thousand times more destructive to living tissue than cyanide

This chapter will further explore cell damage caused by free radicals. This is essential to understanding the aging process and how to slow it down. Free radicals are molecules that react readily with other biological materials. Do not worry about cell phone damage— free radicals are some of the strongest chemical and biological poisons on the planet, and their danger far outweighs cell phone risks.

I emphasize this claim because many doctors and members of the public still do not appreciate the poisonous nature of free radicals. Ask any trained chemist or physicist, and they immediately grasp their toxic significance and admit the hard truth. Free radicals and their byproducts, peroxides, are continually being generated in the body as a normal part of oxygen metabolism. Their huge reactivity makes them a thousand times more destructive to living tissue than *cyanide*, a surprising fact usually not known or believed by many who cling to their dearest illusions.

Free radicals are generated in enormous quantities by all organisms that burn oxygen, and they are cascading prolifically 24/7.

The Scientific Explanation

The Superoxide Anion Radical and Cell Damage
Superoxide has a relatively long lifespan in the fluid of our body's cells relative to other free radicals. Its longevity allows it to wander about helter-skelter in the interior of our cells causing havoc.

Often, the most damaging free radicals generated in the body are the superoxide anion radicals symbolized by $O2^-\bullet$. As previously stated, an exact percentage of all oxygen we consume diverts itself to superoxide production. Fortunately, most of this superoxide becomes inactivated by the enzyme SOD or *superoxide dismutase, a powerful first line of defense in primates,* but not found in most other species. Superoxide has a relatively *long lifespan* in the fluid of your body's cells relative to other free radicals. Its longevity allows it to wander about helter-skelter in the interior of your cells causing havoc and damage, especially to your DNA. It is implicated in some forms of cancer, atherosclerosis, and alcohol-induced liver damage. This latter damage indicates why alcoholics age much faster than the normal population.

We can thank evolution for other lines of defense that prevent DNA damage, particularly mitochondrial DNA damage. In the case of life-threatening ischemia and stroke, superoxide probably remains responsible. *Other mammals lacking the enzyme SOD have shortened lifespans.* For example, my Jack Russell terrier, Algot lacks SOD, but if he had it, he would live longer than his fifteen-to-seventeen-year biological clock. If SOD could be added to his genes, Algot would live to forty in good health. But instead of reprogramming his DNA, we can strengthen his lines of defense with efficient free-radical scavengers and adjust for any hormonal deficiencies.

Healthy Living beyond Age 40 in spite of
Free Radicals, Heavy Exercise, Sports, and Meth Drugs
People over fifty who engage in heavy aerobic exercise
and refuse to take efficient scavenger therapy will experience rapid
whitening of their hair, wrinkled skin, tissue damage, and many
other aging phenomena.

As a teenager my mother continually badgered me to get out in the sunshine and acquire a nice "healthy" tan like my sisters. Today, I have incredibly healthy skin while my sisters' skin has become wrinkled by the free radicals generated by solar radiation from many decades ago. My mother also hassled me about becoming more active in aerobic sports. I loved to exercise, but usually in non-aerobic sports such as sailing, light swimming and biking, and walking. I did not know it then, but non-aerobic sports kept me in shape while only marginalizing free-radical damage caused by breathing. Damage originates from superoxides in *heavy*, aerobic exercise. In this instance I define ***heavy aerobic exercise*** to mean heavy muscular use which thrusts the chest to vigorously expand and contract and forces the lungs to injest large volumes of oxygen.

As mentioned in Chapter 2, my original research indicates that *eight times* the normal amount of superoxides is generated during heavy aerobic exercise versus a resting state. This eightfold increase means that our vital *SOD line of defense* is overwhelmed, and superoxide radicals freely wander about our cells and body causing havoc. Fortunately, other lines of defense using vitamins, glutathione, and other free-radical scavengers can deactivate *some* of these excesses, but not all of them. Damage happens, and it *accumulates over decades of aging* in what medical scientists call micro-insults. During periods of less than one year, damage may even occur very rapidly if one engages in heavy aerobic exercise without taking ***very strong and efficient*** free-radical scavengers; simply using vitamins will not fully address the problem. This unfortunate situation may become further aggravated by hormonal deficiencies, especially a lack of thyroid, testosterone, estradiol, progesterone, oxytocin, melatonin, and growth hormones.

My new research shows that drug addicts using *methamphetamine* incur a similar eightfold excess of free-radicals, and this causes a great

deal of damage. If you doubt this statement, please c
wrinkled, gaunt, and whitened faces of heavy meth users. C
aerobic sports do not have the same degree of negative conse
as methamphetamine addiction, but in a limited way those ada   ⌄
aerobic sports will pay *some* of the same price biologically as those
addicted to meth.

Therefore, please exercise religiously at least thirty minutes
daily, but try to avoid *heavy* aerobic exercise and speed drugs if
you wish to avoid cellular damage resulting from free radicals and
consequent aging. Optimally, one should exercise non-aerobically
with large muscle groups at least one and one half hours daily
since in younger people heavy exercise provides substantial
increases in testosterone, cortisol, and growth hormones. On the
other hand, when people exercise over the age of 50, they only
generate marginal amounts of hormones due to shrunken
endocrine glands. Consequently, the young and especially the old
should protect themselves and consume during heavy exercise
truly STRONG and EFFICIENT free-radical scavengers and fix
any hormonal imbalances. Beware.

**My original research indicates that people over fifty who
engage in heavy aerobic exercise and refuse to take efficient
scavenger therapy will experience rapid whitening of their hair,
wrinkled skin, tissue damage, and many other aging phenomena.
Hair whitening and deepening nasolabial folds** (deep grooves on
the sides of the nose and mouth) **are the strongest indicators of
aging.** These adverse indicators may be viewed in many photos from
an excellent book called *Body for Life* by Bill Phillips, 2008.

Consider that non-aerobic daily exercise is common in Europe
and Japan and frequently takes the form of walking several hours
daily. Long walks easily fulfill health requirements of regular, non-
aerobic exercise since this method employs large muscle groups to
the best advantage. Tennis and swimming are two others. All
Americans should do as their European and Japanese cousins.

Sports-minded friends of mine have questioned my assertion that
they should avoid heavy aerobic exercise. I respond by asking them
to name famous athletes, listing them according to their participation
in *heavy* aerobic versus non-aerobic sports. Guess what? All of the
athletes who lived normal lifespans between 75 and 85 years

participated in sports such as swimming, tennis, or golfing, while those with shortened lifespans played heavy aerobic sports. Of the latter, Jesse Owens comes to mind, a multiple Olympic gold winner who died at the early age of 68. Others include such notables as Joe Louis, Sugar Ray Robinson, Jackie Robinson, and Babe Didrickson – *All of whom died prematurely from natural causes in their sixties or even earlier, and none of whom had serious sports injuries that would account for their shortened lives.*

Shortened lives are common in India where ordinary *vegetarian* laborers work very hard aerobically and die on average at age 55. On the other hand, overweight Indian money-lenders who sit all day and count money die on average at age 75 like most Westerners. Heavy physical labor burns up a body. Make no mistake.

My special research has concluded the following: A shortened lifespan remains a consequence of playing *heavy* aerobic sports or working a *heavy* manual job. This functions somewhat the same way as drug-addicted people who shorten their lives with speed. But there may be understandable lapses. Some tortoises in the Galapagos Islands and in New England live to over 150 years since their free radicals become limited due to their hibernating at low body temperatures and not consuming large quantities of oxygen and producing large amounts of free radicals. At the other extreme, researchers in the Biology Department at Southern Methodist University noted that old male fruit flies put in a cage with young female flies *heavily* exercise themselves to an early death by copulation! Free radicals generated by their flapping wings literally burned them up and wore them out before their time. I can only hope that my readers will heed this warning and exercise due diligence when consorting with younger members of the opposite sex!

The Scientific Explanation #2

Preventing Damages from Radiation which Causes the Short-Lived Hydroxyl Radical
If physicians and dentists understood the type of cellular damage caused by radiation, they may not be so cavalier about its routine use.

A second extremely powerful toxin that plagues humanity is the *hydroxyl free radical*. Generally speaking, when generated inside the cells of the body, it reacts with the first available molecule it contacts, namely water which forms new free radicals. This is caused by its limited *nanosecond lifespan*, and therefore it lacks the time to wander about the cell's interior and do damage like superoxide. Only physicists with extremely sensitive detectors tied to oscilloscopes have accurately measured this nanosecond activity.

A further proof of its short nanosecond lifespan I have drawn from Mother Nature herself: *She refuses to provide living organisms with enzymes or lines of defense that deactivate hydroxyl radicals, as She has done with the longer-lived superoxide.* This basic fact explains why both nuclear radiation and normal aging damage our health. Short-lived hydroxyl radicals cause declines in health, and we remain without enzymatic defenses against them. However, intervention with anti-radiation nutrients will deactivate them. Thus, I consume *l-methionine, l-acetyl cysteine,* and l-*glutathione* or BHT daily, 250 mg with each meal. My own radical-scavenger formulation registered with the Swedish and Italian FDAs is called ACF228. This is my new and special research which enhances our health and adds years to our lives and life to our years.

But there is one exception. If a powerful beam of gamma radiation irradiates our cells, then hydroxyl radicals *cascade* in abundance and quickly damage everything in proximity. This only occurs in a nuclear blast, or from a CAT scan, whole-body scan, or an x-ray machine. Thus, I personally refuse them; including x-ray scans from dentists or physicians, except in the event of an emergency. If physicians and dentists understood the type of cellular damage caused by radiation, they may not be so cavalier about its routine use. No one should routinely accept radiation in their mouth, head, or chest. I do not understand this "routine dental x-ray" mentality. When I know that I must be x-rayed, I always consume radio-protective nutrients an hour in advance. For example, two grams of effective free-radical scavengers such as l-methionine, *l*-acetyl-cysteine, penicillamine, ACF228, and l-glutathione do nicely in mopping-up hydroxyl and other radicals.

Special Free-Radical Scavengers Employed for Better Health
During WWII, American soldiers were given K-rations laced with the food preservative BHT, and their rate of stomach cancer dropped by one third!

Free-radical scavengers are materials like green tea that becomes oxidized to black tea when oxygen attaches itself to chemically sensitive green-tea molecules, and we visualize this process by noticing a darkening in tea color. Thus, green tea and other scavenger materials inside our bodies have the potential to deactivate and prevent damage to organic molecules inside our skin, organs, and tissues of our bodies. Other common free-radical scavengers are the *anthocyanins* found in red wine that stabilize it and protect it from turning orange. We also find them naturally included in our diets in small concentrations such as Vitamins C and E, and sulphur-amino acids. Some synthetic free-radical scavengers added are the food additives *sodium benzoate* and BHT or *butylated hydroxy toluene*, which are many orders of magnitude stronger than these vitamins, and help to preserve our food as well as our bodies. Case in point: During WWII, American soldiers were given K-rations laced with BHT, and their rate of stomach cancer dropped by one third!

Mother Nature's Defenses are often useless against Active Oxygens
Human lines of defense only need a minor lifting up by the boot straps with my one-meal one-pill regimen combined with some depleted hormones.

Many people do not understand that Mother Nature has provided living creatures with enzymes to deactivate superoxide free radicals and hydrogen peroxide. On the other hand, *active-oxygen species* such as hydroxyl free radicals and *singlet oxygen* have no deactivating enzymes in living organisms since they only exist for nanoseconds. Another type of active oxygen called singlet oxygen is defined as a hyper-activated state of the oxygen molecule. This is only reasonable and logical but often misunderstood.

To counter micro-insults to your body, I avoid mountains of pills.

namely the critical postmitotic or non-replicating cells of the heart, brain, and central nervous system. If you enjoy your life and health for decades to come, this specific anti-aging therapy is priceless, especially if combined with hormone replacement and anti-cross linking therapies. At age 63 I have skin and internal organs of a youngster due to my one pill/one meal regimen of truly *strong* free-radical scavengers, anti-cross linkers, and bio-identical hormones. My typical blood pressure is 118 over 60 which usually only young people have. Medical studies report that average human blood pressure is 115 over 75, while the blood pressure in a giraffe is typically 250 over 150 mm mercury due to their long necks.

Please observe that the lifespans of dogs, rats, mice, and chickens increased up to 50% by supplementing *strong* free-radical scavengers as first suggested by Professor Denham Harman's revolutionary work in 1956. Then he proved in the early 1980's that *mega-dosing* with large handfuls of scavengers or antioxidants do not work. Indeed, large handfuls of antioxidants can turn them into *pro-oxidants* and increase our rate of aging. Our lab animals did attain huge boosts in longevity with moderate therapy even though they lack the efficient lines of defense that humans possess. *Human lines of defense only need a minor lifting up by the boot straps with my one-meal one-pill regimen combined with some depleted hormones and anti-cross linkers.*

My measuring with unique instruments helps to lower free radicals, increase metabolic efficiency, and slow aging at the cellular and tissue levels. The rewards of my therapies will be quite dramatic if you later compare yourself with your contemporaries in the coming decades. You decide. For me, taking one pill with every meal for the last three decades has been a slam dunk.

Further Thoughts on Radicals and Our Protection
Humans could be enhanced with boosted lines of defense against free radicals—especially the DNA of our mitochondria where most free radicals are generated and the damage most crucial.

Currently, anti-aging research can extend lifespan, health, and memory far beyond the traditional bounds of the Bible's three score and ten (70) years. I believe active and healthy centenarians can become the norm, not the exception, in the near future if anti-aging medicine were implemented. More dramatic results like a doubling of lifespan demand far more detailed knowledge of cellular biology. This is invitingly close at hand, and among scientists like me the excitement has become enormous. In this regard, I believe research into gene and hormone therapies hold the most promise. These therapies have not yet impacted medicine significantly. For example, the natural, bio-identical hormone *progesterone* turns on the *p53 gene* which in turn inhibits cancers of the breast and prostate.

In regard to added protection from free radicals, I am hopeful that a younger generation of researchers will begin to explore the modification of the human genome with the introduction of new genetic materials known to increase our natural lines of defense against free radicals. I can also hope that hormone researchers will soon discover how to better control our metabolisms with fewer prescription drugs, and some leading anti-aging physicians have achieved that in their medical practices. For example, in animal-research dogs could live to age forty and cats to fifty if their genomes were enhanced, and hormones balanced. Humans could also boost themselves with increased enzymatic lines of defense against free radicals—especially in mitochondrial DNA where most free radicals and damages are generated. Another genetic advance might increase hormone producing cells and reverse the atrophy of our endocrine glands after middle-age. Lastly, enhancing stem cells and reducing *telomere* (gene) damages will probably become the next decade's advancements in longevity. Already some telomere damages have been limited due to a recent remedy call the "Patton Protocol."

What is the timetable for the above advances in anti-aging? Medical knowledge doubles every five or six years, and some anti-aging physicians have predicted that by the year 2026 all major diseases will be cured or curable. If we can only live another twenty years and not deteriorate too rapidly with the aid of today's technologies, a new lease on life awaits us. The Irish critic and playwright George Bernard Shaw once said: "Some men see things as they are and ask why. Others dream things that never were and ask why not." I always ask why not, and you should too.

Recommendations

- Drink filtered or **glass**-bottled water: Pollutants in our environment contribute to aging. • For emergency x-rays, consume 2 grams l-methionine or l-glutathione. Consume 50 mg/d l-glutathione and more with a high fresh-fish diet. Also use 3X daily with meals 250 mg/d min. l-methionine, l-cysteine, or l-acetyl cysteine. Take minimum 50 mg/d BHT, BHA, or ACF 228. www.antiaging-motivate.com Wash everything down with grapefruit or pomegranate juices diluted in filtered water..
- Exercise minimum 30 min/d non-aerobically, such as walking, golfing, light biking, and playing tennis. 1½ hours of non-aerobic exercise daily is preferable, especially if combined with efficient free-radical scavengers with every meal.

Golden Keys to Longevity #4

- *Since our lines of defense against poisonous free radicals become overwhelmed by eight times the normal with heavy aerobic exercise, it is critical to consume judicious amounts of strong and effective free-radical scavengers with every meal and maintain balanced hormones. A shortened lifespan remains a consequence of playing heavy aerobic sports or working a heavy manual job somewhat like drug-addicted people shorten their lives with speed. These are my new and unique research conclusions.*

End Notes: [1]*Nature*, 2006 Apr 13:440(7086), pp. 944-948. Dig Dis Sci 2007 Sep 52(9), pp. 2015-2021. Free Radic Biol Med 2008 Apr 15; 44(8), pp.1493-1505. Proc Nutr Soc 2008 May; 67(2), pp.214-222.

Chapter 5
Will Death Be Optional?

Live 60 Frank Sinatra Years Instead Of 100 Spiro Agnew Years?
*"It's time to get the performance-enhancing drugs out of baseball
and back where they belong—in some octogenarian's testicles."*
Bill Maher

The scientists and I gathered in comforting leather armchairs in front of a crackling fireplace. A heated debate raged before the smoldering logs and acrid smoke. Some of us believed that we were still destined to die the "old fashion way"—Alzheimer's, cancer, and heart disease. In contrast, others believed that ushering in a new slowed-aging epoch would happen only by following a strict anti-aging regimen. The old fashion way could only be defeated by enhancements in genes, hormone replacement, stem cells, organ cloning, *strong* antioxidants and anti-cross linkers.

Then I noticed something strange.

Two of the scientists who were advocating the "old fashion way" were the same age of 66, and they looked it, namely white hair, wrinkled melting faces, and turkey-necks. One had dark pigmentation under reddening eyelids which betrayed weak adrenal glands. Another showed excessive nose hair indicative of low progesterone. These are typical symptoms of raging biological aging.

On the other hand, another 65 year old scientist who argued for intervention with a strict anti-aging regimen appeared to be about 12 years younger. Like me, he had actually practiced anti-aging medicine for many years, and consequently, his hair was thick and only partly grey, his neck was rather smoothed-skin, and his faced betrayed some wrinkles only around the eyes. His adrenals were strong, and the skin on his forearms was especially healthy and youthful.

Using my advice, he took strong free-radical scavengers with every meal and bio-identical replacement of natural testosterone, melatonin, HGH, and thyroid hormones. Indeed, natural testosterone cream had significantly impacted his aging and age-related problems instead of using drugs. (See *New England Journal of Medicine*, Dec. 2007, Vol.357, No. 24, pp. 2472-2481) He looked great at 65 or even if he had been 50, and I was struck by the dramatic contrast between him and the two others. Biological and chronological age can diverge from each other if one follows a constructive anti-aging plan.

With these significant differences in mind, I began to contemplate how others could slow their aging on a practical level. The first step is to read and understand the clinical double-blind evidence from leading medical journals as cited above. The second step is to ignore all the nay-Sayers from academia stuck in their orthodoxies and traditions. The following is one such sad story of outdated attitudes.

Anti-aging medicine is repeatedly discounted by some misguided academics from prestigious medical schools despite the mounting evidence of its scientific veracity. A general lack of awareness prevails concerning those with aging problems, and especially those who are hormonally challenged. Several years ago, one such academic was paid a large advance from a publisher to investigate and write about aging and anti-aging. He understood nutrition and diet, and only armed with this knowledge set forth to a convention of the American Academy of Anti-Aging Medicine. One would have hoped that he would approach this conference with an open mind, attend the lectures of prominent physicians practicing anti-aging medicine, and lastly examine the scientific references of all claims made. He refused. Instead of attending lectures, he headed for the exhibition hall where he discovered small companies hyping a variety of nutritional products, many of which with weak scientific claims. On this basis, he dismissed any idea that real anti-aging medicine and therapy even existed.

Attacking the Source of One's Aging Problems

Unfortunately such bias holds sway over the American public, leaving them to spend their time and money on plastic surgery, temporary cosmetic remedies, and other superficial stop-gap measures instead of attacking the source of our aging problems. For example, did you know that a coronary bypass is universally acknowledged as a *band-aid approach* to heart disease? Any surgeon will tell you that bypass *only* oxygenates the heart with the insertion of extra band aid-like blood vessels, while the remaining arteries in the body continue to become clogged with fat until they choke off your body's supply of oxygen and nutrients and eventually kill you. But lacking monetary incentives, these same surgeons ignore the alternatives, namely known methods to repair and revitalize all of the body's aging arteries.

My Personal Anti-Aging Story
I sought ways to intercede with a wide array of hormone therapies applied in anti-aging medicine.

My family story of anti-aging medicine began in 1978. I was married to a beautiful and intelligent Swedish girl with long blonde hair who had a history of fashion modeling in Paris. We had a happy household with two tow-headed babies. Then one evening I arrived home from my research lab to discover my lovely wife lying on the bed with her hands pressed to her chest. "What am I going to do," she exclaimed. "My heart beats like a sludge hammer. I am going to die," she kept repeating. She had visited numerous physicians without a proper diagnosis while her appearance and health deteriorated. I questioned her more closely and asked about the physical appearance of her mother just before her untimely death eight years previously. Her mother also had a racing heartbeat, and at the time of her death she had bulging eyes as evidenced by old photos. These were classic symptoms of *hyperthyroidism* characterized by excessive amounts of thyroid hormone circulating in the body. I told my wife my suspicions, and had her see a qualified endocrinologist. She visited several until finally one of them confirmed my diagnoses and treated her. What a relief when my wife's medical crisis resolved itself by using hormone therapy.

Realizing how a hormonal imbalance had affected my wife's health, aging and appearance, I resolved to learn more about hormones and their effects upon the aging process. I began to read every research paper available on hormones, their proper balance, and how an imbalance would adversely affect longevity. In 1978, my medical professors stated that hormone imbalances and a shortened lifespan were inevitable. The most obvious example I found in the case of diabetics who lack the hormone insulin, and must inject themselves daily. If diabetics stop monitoring their blood sugar or stop their daily injections, they become ill and their lifespans are shortened. As a consequence, I sought ways to intercede with a wide array of hormone therapies applied in anti-aging medicine. Eventually my research achieved some minor new advances in hormone treatment.

Some Basic Facts about Hormones
Hormone reinstatement to younger levels and avoiding synthetic drugs is one of many exceptional methods of addressing aging.

Hormones control everything in the body, especially organs and individual cells. Our hormones are inherited from our ancestors. Unknown to many, male and females have the same number of hormones, but in different concentrations. Lastly and most importantly in regard to aging, hormone levels decrease as we age with few exceptions. These decreases are directly responsible for many of our symptoms of aging. Thus, hormone reinstatement to younger levels is one of many exceptional methods of addressing aging.

Remarkable Alternatives to Standard Surgery
or Drug Approaches
Anti-aging therapy using testosterone in the case of men and other vital hormones and nutrients in the case of women can dramatically affect the aging of hearts and arteries.

Alternatives to hormonal deficiencies, surgery and statin drugs do exist. These include the aforementioned nutrient aminoguanidine, and by examining the practices of a remarkable Danish physician, Jens Møller, MD (pronounced "Yens Mer-ler."). In Copenhagen, Denmark, Dr. Møller and his colleagues cured patients with cardiovascular disease, or *CVD*, for over forty years. CVD is a form of *accelerated aging* like Type 2 diabetes, and it remains very relevant to the aging process since over 40% of the American population will die from heart disease, and approximately 80% of these deaths will occur between the ages of 65 and 100. Mark my words; CVD is extremely relevant to your future health and longevity.

Dr. Møller conclusively demonstrated that many deleterious effects of CVD are slowed or even reversed with hormone treatment. During a forty year period of medical practice, he helped thousands of patients with typical CVD problems such as chest pains, angina, cardiac ischemia (narrowed blood vessels), myocardial infarction (heart attack), and claudication (peripheral vascular disease).

His remarkable treatments existed long before statin drugs were invented and endlessly touted by the pharmaceutical industry. This industry has a vested interest in *patented* medications that make them profits and are needed by *some* patients. However, most patients should use more natural remedies, especially bio-identical testosterone replacement. This vital point is often ignored by the status quo of the medical community since natural remedies lack profit, and cannot be commercially protected by patents.

Dr. Møller employed one of Mother Nature's most powerful tools to combat CVD, the natural hormone testosterone. This treatment made him a pioneer in hormone replacement therapy as early as 1948. He would often inject 250 mg *testosterone enanthate* three times weekly in only male patients suffering CVD, and he and his colleagues documented dramatic improvements in over 80% of the cases thus treated. Employing this method, arteries regained their health, and clogging with fatty plaques subsided. Health restored itself as Mother Nature had intended with a natural substance.

The most significant results were seen in patients with *gangrene* who other physicians had abandoned with recommendations for amputating an appendage. *Gangrene is accelerated aging of the arteries when they lose their ability to oxygenate tissues*, which become purple and black from necrosis, or cell death. *The progressive healing of gangrene tissue clearly demonstrates that anti-aging therapy can dramatically affect aging of the heart and arteries.* Testosterone repairs arteries in the case of men, while other related hormones are used in the case of women. Believe it. Maintenance of healthy arteries and tissues long into your 80's and 90's becomes truly possible with bio-identical hormone replacement therapy. Women especially need replacement of their unique deficiencies by balancing bio-identical estradiol, progesterone, *limited* testosterone, and estriol. I cannot emphasize this point enough. Success with your rate of aging and susceptibility to disease becomes practical with hormone replacement therapy. In other words, do not become hormonally challenged.

Short History of Hormone Replacement
The celestial emperor ordered all young members of his court to separate by sex and urinate daily into two large troughs.

Although ancient Greeks hypothesized the existence of the hormone testosterone, the first recorded use of hormones started in the first century AD by wealthy Roman women. Like 40% of American women today, these women suffered from sexual dysfunction. Consequently, these Roman women purchased expensive oils harvested from scraping the bodies of male gladiators and applying harvested oils to their genitals. In 2002, a study from University of California at Berkeley tested similar oils gathered from the bodies of male athletes and found them to contain the testosterone metabolite *androstenediene*. Further testing with female student volunteers revealed an increase in the hormone cortisone and perhaps even other testosterone metabolites.

Beginning in the 11th century, the Chinese were second in the use of bio-identical hormone replacement from 1025 AD to 1833 AD. In Beijing, the Chinese called their emperor's palace *"celestial heaven"* since they believed that nothing worthwhile was created outside of this sacred place. The celestial emperor ordered all young members of his court to separate by sex and urinate daily into two large troughs. The emperor's pharmacy staff collected urine daily, and they harvested urinary salts by precipitating them with saponifyng or soap-like chemicals. Then they further isolated and harvested bio-identical hormones (*chhiu shih*) which were rolled together in the shape of small resin balls and distributed to the emperor and his empress according to their male or female origin. Other aging members of the celestial palace received and used left-over resin balls. This unique therapy resulted in enhanced health and longevity to China's ruling elite, which inadvertently may have contributed to the development of some remarkable inventions in ancient China, namely gunpowder, canons, rockets, ink, paper, and the printing press. That is what I call bio-identical hormone replacement.

Centuries later in Merry Olde England during the time of Shakespeare, Englishmen consumed food containing hormone-rich glands. For example in English kitchens at the beginning of every week, housewives baked their meat pies and inserted *sweat meats* or kidney and thyroid glands from pigs and birds. Thus, this quaint custom was probably the origin of the old English song, "Four and twenty black birds baked in a pie." It also attested to the wisdom of the Greek physician, Hippocrates who wrote "Let food be your medicine and medicine be your food."

Unlike present-day English meat pies, these 17th century pie crusts were never eaten since they were only used as ecological packaging material. By *lightly* baking the meat pies, the sweat meats remained somewhat raw inside, and thus biologically viable and rich in natural hormones, especially in the case of pig thyroid glands containing the highly active thyroid hormone, T3. Thyroid hormones sustain our health and prevent hypothyroidism.

In addition to the consumption of semi-raw endocrine glands, housewives added raw cock's comb to their meat pies. In today's modern world, cock's comb remains the richest known source of *hyaluronic acid.* This acid naturally retains moisture in our skin since it absorbs about eight times its weight in water. Dermatologists routinely inject it in the lower half of their patient's faces to insure a more youthful and fresh appearance. When injected into the lip line, it radiates with a special brilliance from reflective light. Apparently, in past centuries Englishmen enhanced their skin by eating semi-raw cock's comb rich in hyaluronic acid. When my modern-day patients experimented by consuming 6 capsules daily of 8% hyaluronic acid, their skin became shinier after a few months. Nothing like obtaining radiant skin the natural way without using expensive cosmetic creams or painful injections! Hyaluronic acid fortifies and beautifies our skin much like the car-care product, Amoral® adds shine and freshness to an automobile's tires and vinyl interiors. Try them sometime.

Thanks to the Romans, Chinese, and English, natural bio-identical hormones made their impact on health and longevity many centuries before the pharmaceutical industry synthesized and patented "space-alien drug-hormones." This later phrase means that in a never-ending quest for profits, the pharmaceutical industry chooses to synthesize *analogs* to natural hormones which they could commercially protect by patents instead of merely selling natural hormones that cannot be patented and therefore are unprofitable. Here again I am not against the capitalist system which has been enormously beneficial in this country. I am merely stating that because of the current patent system in place, space-alien drug-hormones are often being promoted when natural hormones or other nutrients would be more beneficial. Back to hormone history.

In 1849 the German physiologist Arnold Berthold produced secondary sexual characteristics in immature cocks by surgically attaching the testicles of mature cocks. This was also the first formal therapeutic test of hormones in the Western world since the cock's comb increased in size due to the stimulation of attached testicles. During World War I, the famous Danish surgeon Thorkild Rovsing attached the testicles of a newly deceased soldier onto an old patient with gangrene. The gangrene healed completely, and the first proof of testosterone's positive effects upon the circulatory system was demonstrated. Then in 1931, researchers Adolf Butenandt and Kurt Tscherning in Göttingen, Germany succeeded in isolating 50 mg of pure crystalline *androsterone*, an estrone metabolite from testosterone. In 1934 they discovered the formula for testosterone for which they received the Nobel Prize in Chemistry the following year. Up into the 1940's, doctor Paul Niehans developed the first cellular therapies with injections of fetal animal cells into humans to rejuvenate weak and failing organs and tissues of aging patients.

Background of Hormones and Their Use in America
His research laid the groundwork for our understanding of how cortisol works in humans and how to best administer it in cases of deficiency.

In 1937, we encounter the remarkable research of ophthalmologist and Columbia University affiliated, Dr. Emanuel Josephson. His research revealed a cause of some eye problems called glaucomas. These patients suffered from hypoadrenalism (weak adrenal glands), and their damaged adrenals induced *glaucoma*. Acting on this premise, he made extracts called *ACE* or *Cortin* from cattle adrenals, and injected these extracts into glaucoma suffers. Many patients were dramatically improved as evidenced by the lowering of intra-ocular pressures of their eyes.

Subsequently, in 1948 endocrinologist Dr. William Jeffries received a small quantity of the newly isolated hormone *cortisol*, which is known today to be one of the most biologically active hormones produced by adrenal glands. He studied cortisol for over thirty years with numerous patients, and his research laid the groundwork for our understanding of how cortisol works in humans and how to best administer it in cases of deficiency. Too much or too little results in greatly increased risk of infections and inflammations. Thus, exact dosages that properly balance all hormones have always been advisable.

The Man Who Brought Reproductive Freedom and Longevity to American Women
Is it any wonder that women would eventually turn to hormonal replacement methods proven in Europe?

Until the introduction of birth control pills in the late 1950s, American women had no reproductive freedom. They could not "just say no" to their husbands' sexual advances, despite what some American politicos may tell you. Pregnancies were often unplanned, and many American women died prematurely before what we label today as middle age. In other words, when a woman gave birth nearly every year during her young adulthood, she could not expect long life, nor could she expect adequate post-menopausal medical care.

Enter the renowned pharmacist, my dear friend James Jamieson, who has sparkling eyes, a warm smile, and friendly attitude. Jim first brought bio-identical, birth-control pills to America from Italy in 1956. The raw materials of these pills were extracted from yams and compressed into tablets. Yams have been known for decades as a concentrated source of natural hormones that could be chemically extracted and purified with chromatography. The true breakthrough came in 1943 when Professor Russell Marker of the University of Pennsylvania visited Mexico. He discovered that local shaman had used an extracted white powder from Barbasco yams for centuries for birth control and the treatment of female problems. Mexican farmers grew yams in mountain underground gardens much like potatoes. When Marker returned to the U.S., he had his bag of white powder analyzed and discovered that it contained highly purified *progesterone*, a hormone essential for proper health, especially in women. The pharmaceutical giant Upjohn eventually employed Dr. Marker's superior purification techniques. This remarkable work provided me with one of many reasons why I recommend 100 mg progesterone daily for women who desire hormonal balance and longevity. Over 40 men should only use 15 to 30 mg daily.

Subsequently, in 1951 Fortune Magazine wrote that yam harvesting had created a minor Mexican agricultural boom with much of the harvest shipped to Europe. In the US, the Jamieson's family chain of drug stores sold these yam extracts during the late

1950s. Jamieson's importation, manufacturing, and sale of birth-control pills unknowingly created a steady platform for the women's liberation movement of the 1960s. Before birth control, middle-class women in past centuries were pregnant between seven and twenty-two times during their lifetimes. While brilliant men contemplated solutions to humanity's problems, women occupied themselves with feeding hungry mouths and wiping behinds. Bravo for Jim. In later years, he brought to America a cheaper version of Librium® and many other remarkable medications since the existing U.S. versions were ridiculously expensive and difficult to obtain.

I first met Jim Jamieson in 1988 at the offices of The Journal of Longevity in Marina del Rey, California. He knew that I had invented the nicotine patch as well as diet patches during the preceding four years. Jim wanted me to experiment with a hormone patch since such an invention would be a quick and efficient method to help people with hormone deficiencies. I toyed with the idea in my laboratory and developed a patch soaked with thyroxine or thyroid hormone. But unfortunately, we discovered that it violated the law since many hormones are strictly controlled by prescription. At the time, pharmaceutical companies were uninterested for sundry reasons, but it is still a great idea whose time has yet to come. Allow me to add, however, that many hormones are quite rightly restricted by our FDA since hormones are extremely *powerful* substances, and their use is only advisable under the supervision of knowledgeable medical professionals. Interestingly, most drug companies have no real interest in promoting them since they are unpatentable and thus not profitable.

Another true pioneer in the field of glandular and hormonal extracts was a genius doctor named Arthur Karler. He apprenticed to a famous German-Jewish medical doctor who had moved south of the border, to Mexico, in the aftermath of the Holocaust in Germany. In the 1920s, German and Swiss doctors had successfully used extracts in their medical practice as evidenced by doctors Paul Niehans, Paul T. Urol, and Henry Harrower. This unnamed German-Jewish doctor exhibited a distinctly Teutonic manner since he wore a monocle and shaved his head much like the filmmaker, Erich von Stroheim. During the 1950's their border-town clinic in northern Mexico employed hormone extracts from animal sources that were largely outlawed in the U.S. Their border-town clinic helped thousands of Americans who could not receive proper therapy at home since conventional American medicine and law refused to allow organ extracts and hormone therapy. This miserable law violating freedom of choice was finally changed in 2003.

Interestingly, the above violation of free choice existed despite the work of Dr. G. Roth of the Mayo Clinic who reported in 1933 that pancreatic tissue extract was "the only substance now known which has definite and striking effect on symptoms of 'intermittent claudication," or cramp-like pains in the calves caused by poor blood circulation. Why cannot we trust are best scientists in this country?

My mother, Kay Lippman, R.N., needed help with her hormones during the 1950s, and her doctors ignored her problems and shrugged off her symptoms as "female delusions." In the 1930s women were sometimes given shock therapy to "cure" their hormonal deficiencies. Is it any wonder that women would eventually turn to hormonal replacement methods proven in Europe?

Another more dramatic example involves the medical history of President John F. Kennedy. Kennedy suffered terribly during his short life since he had Addison's disease which means a lack of hormones such as cortisol originating from his adrenal glands. If Kennedy had survived his assassination and lived today, his disease would have been remedied during the last few decades with natural hormone replacement therapy.

An Intriguing Case History of Hormone Replacement Therapy
He heard rumors of the thousands of Americanos who visit the town seeking medical help.

Allow me to inject an amusing case history related to me by my friend Dr. Arthur Karler. Dr. Karler and his German-Jewish mentor had no medical or business license to practice medicine in a small Mexican border town. One day the President of Mexico, called "El Presidente", arrived in this small border town and acquired lodgings in the town's best hotel. Dr. Karler felt unglued since as a result of El Presidente's arrival, he might well be arrested for a lack of the necessary licenses needed to practice in Mexico. Finally, he summoned up some courage and boldly marched himself to the front desk of El Presidente's hotel. Dr. Karler asked the desk clerk to ring the suite of El Presidente. The trembling desk clerk flatly refused. Eventually the hotel manager intervened and arranged an audience with El Presidente. Taking the bull by the horns, Dr. Karler took the elevator upstairs and respectfully approached El Presidente. El Presidente smiled warmly, and the two men shook hands. Then surprisingly El Presidente congratulated Dr. Karler for bringing prosperity to this small Mexican border town! Apparently El Presidente had heard rumors of the thousands of *Americanos* who visited the town seeking medical help. He also asked Dr. Karler for help concerning his own medical problems which would be diagnosed today as chronic fatigue syndrome. Dr. Karler happily obliged with an "*ACE Booster*" based on the research of the eminent endocrinologist Emanuel Josephson. During his week-long visit, El Presidente gained in strength and energy, and he and Dr. Karler became fast friends. Also, from that day forward the local Mexican police treated Dr. Karler with respect since he was the amigo of El Presidente! I wonder if Presidente Calderón is equally amiable to American enterprise in Mexico today despite border and NAFTA conflicts?

Let us continue with our story. Dr. Karler developed special hormonal and thymic extracts from cattle organs that would aid patients suffering from a myriad of diagnosed and undiagnosed endocrine problems. These extracts stimulate the immune system and aid in wound healing. Eventually, when some restrictive American laws changed, Dr. Karler made custom extracts in the U.S. from various slaughterhouse organs which he labeled "ACE Boosters," using techniques learned from Dr. Emanuel Josephson's pioneering research. He published his beneficial and revolutionary work in the Britain's foremost medical journal, *Nature,* in 1961. Then during the 1970's, endocrinologist Dr. John Tintera focused his research on adrenal gland weaknesses found in Addison's disease (a collapse of the adrenal gland). He began advocating whole adrenal gland extracts and not isolated steroid hormones or patented pseudo or space-alien steroids. As a result of his whole-organ therapy, he was formally expelled from the New York Medical Society.

Beginning in the 1970's, Dr. John R. Lee, a true pioneer in using bio-identical progesterone, wrote the first prescriptions for thousands of California women for their hot flashes, night sweats, and insomnia. He coined the phrase "*estrogen dominant*" indicating that women lacked *progesterone* and had excessive *estrogens*. After Lee's untimely death, my friend Dr. Jonathan Wright, MD, carried on his work and was responsible for reviving and further popularizing the use of bio-identical estrogens and progesterone. Wright's unique development of the "triple estrogen" or "*Triest* and double estrogen or "*Biest*" formulas have been a godsend to American women suffering menopausal problems. These formulas are completely natural, and thus, they avoid the problems of synthetic hormones, especially increased incidence of cancer, bone loss, and heart problems.

In the late 80's, Genentech manufactured its first recombinant DNA product, human growth hormone or HGH in Stockholm, Sweden. To this day, the highly advanced Swedes sell *over-the-counter* both the hormone *estriol* that prevents breast cancer and the herbal product "*Monks' Pepper*" that alleviates pre-menopausal symptoms. Back in the US, other prescription-only hormones and special recombinant DNA-produced drugs followed such as Genentech's *HGH* and *Avastin®* as well as Amgen's *Enbrel®*. In two recent studies, Enbrel seems to improve cognitive abilities in Alzheimer's patients by over 100%. I strongly favor all of these remarkable American and Swedish products, and I recommend them to everyone seriously interested in an anti-aging regimen.

The arrival of a vast assortment of bio-identical replacement hormones during the last twenty-five years makes hormone and extract therapy practical and available to even those who need supplementation as a result of normal aging. In other words, normal aging can be remedied without any medical risks.

Would You Knowingly Consume Drugs Made from Horse Waste?
He always demonstrated a moral compass in his marketing and did not try to sell horse waste products to the trusting American public.

In dramatic contrast to the above histories are the sad tales of synthetic or space-alien hormones such as methyltestosterone (MT).

Again by "space-alien" I mean designer-drug hormones that are not naturally found in the human body but *synthesized* in a chemical laboratory or perhaps *excreted* from a horse's body. For example, MT was chemically synthesized and administered to millions of men, and it caused angina, liver cancer, and cardiovascular disease. Then other space-aliens were extracted from horse excrement and women were convinced into using it until the release of the bomb-shell Women's Health Initiative Report of 2002. This report said that space-alien hormones were responsible for dramatic increases in breast and cervical cancers. One year after the release of this report, most women realized their mistake and stopped using the space aliens, and subsequently, their rate of cancers dropped by more than half.

Again allow me to state emphatically that I am not an enemy of capitalism or the pharmaceutical industry which I believe has benefitted many Americans. What I am against are irresponsible marketing decisions made by some companies that have led to unfortunate results. For example, at the other extreme I worked for one of America's leading marketers, Glenn Braswell. He always demonstrated a moral compass in his marketing and with significant integrity did not try to sell horse waste products to the trusting American public.

These last two space-aliens, hormones not people, are responsible for needless cancers and a host of other medical problems. The active ingredient medroxyprogesterone is still another example of a space-alien molecule and their downstream metabolites, *4 and 16 alpha hydroxyestrones* which are known and powerful carcinogens. Beware. One would imagine that when Drs. Butenandt and Tscherning won their Nobel Prize for the discovery of testosterone in 1935 that this would have sent a message to the medical community that just maybe natural hormones contribute to good health and longevity. Just maybe.

How Do Hormones Regulate Our Bodies?
Too much or too little of any hormone or if our hormones are unbalanced with one another, then our health greatly suffers.

The glands in our body produce various hormones for the regulation of our organs and cells. For example, the endocrine glands secrete hormones and carry them by the bloodstream to various target organs for their proper control and function. This balancing act is called *homeostasis*, and our bodies must balance themselves with homeostasis to feel well and not rapidly age.

As in the case of free radicals, hormones are extremely powerful substances that critically process and regulate everything in every cell in the body. **Hormone imbalance, or too much or too little of any hormone, results in deteriorating health and aging**. *See Table One. Trying to replace one hormone only without replacing other hormones to match is like shuffling chairs on the Titanic. Avoid it. Replace and balance all hormones together so that they may function in symphony with one another and homeostasis is maintained.*

Over the span of a lifetime imbalances cause shortened lives plagued by a variety of diseases. In other words, hormone imbalances and the cascading of free radicals have significant negative impacts on our patterns of aging. Altered patterns of aging must be medically addressed if we hope to live healthy lives long into the 21st century. Trust me.

Most hormone production declines after age thirty. For example, thyroid hormone declines at least 25-50%, and we really need sufficient thyroid hormones for proper maintenance and homeostasis of body temperature and blood circulation. Some esteemed endocrinologists such as Doctors Jacque and Thierry Hertoghe estimate that 80% of all women over the age of 40 are thyroid deficient. These deficiencies may lead to memory loss, menstrual problems, constipation, cold hands and feet, dry skin, sleep disorders, thinning hair, low energy, weight gain, and an inability to maintain normal metabolism. *Human growth hormone* or HGH declines as much as 90%, and it critically affects our muscle tone, sagging skin, and general health and wellbeing. Indeed, many over the age of ninety have sufficient levels of HGH and another cousin hormone Igf-1. The name "growth hormone" is a misnomer since it does a great deal more than just enable children to grow taller. Furthermore, during aging progesterone production abruptly declines after age 50, and *melatonin* production is cut by two thirds. My own progesterone level declined to one seventh the optimal at age 63, and my testosterone declined to one third the optimal range of values from 750 to 850 ng/dl serum.

In summary, we need these three essential hormones for our libido, sound sleep, smooth skin, and heart and vascular health. Without adequate levels of hormones, we risk death as well as a wide assortment of aliments as depicted in Tables One, Two, and Three.

Your Health and Longevity Critically depend upon Adequate Testosterone and Thyroid Hormones

Tables One and Two below indicate what happens if the two vital hormones, testosterone and thyroid, are deficient. During aging, men reach andropause (male menopause) after age 45. Their female hormones, the estrogens, remain largely unchanged while their testosterone (T) *dramatically decreases* to one third or one fourth of what they had in their 20's or 30's. Thus, due to loss of critical T, the estrogens began to dominate the male body. This means that male bodies become more effeminate with large increases in prostate size, body fat, and sometimes even women's breasts (gynecomastia). This increased body fat produces even more estrogens, and thus, an evil circle of increasing estrogen dominance occurs unopposed by previous high levels of T. This enormous loss offers one reason why men typically live three fewer years on average than women.

Even worse is when these aging men drink cow milk or caffeine drinks. Cow milk contains pseudo-estrogens which add further fuel to the estrogen dominant fire. An ordinary cup of caffeinated coffee temporarily doubles a man's estrogens, and thus further aggravates swollen prostates and urinary problems. Humans are the *only* animals on the planet that drink cow milk and caffeinated drinks. Do not do it if you value your prostate health and longevity.

Women may also become estrogen dominant at any age. Fortunately, Mother Nature provides women with lots of natural *progesterone* to balance and counter the adverse effects of too much estrogen. One exception is when women take the synthetic progesterone alternative, *Provera®* (medroxy-progesterone). Provera alleviates several female problems at the expense of blocking natural progesterone. But instead of getting swollen prostates, women may experience swelling in the embryonic equivalent of the prostate, namely their ovaries and vagina. In fact, when women lack natural

81

progesterone or when it is blocked by synthetic drugs, women are open to uncontrolled cell proliferation or *hyperplasia*. One result may be excessive endometrial bleeding and headaches. Thus, both sexes after menopause and andropause really need at least 20 mg daily of supplemental natural progesterone cream for normal health. Please see further details in Table Three.

Table Two below indicates how one may measure inadequate thyroid hormone at home by taking one's temperature. The best time to take temperature measurements is upon awakening in the morning before breakfast. A second measurement may be warranted if one is inclined to nap in the afternoon or whenever one's hands and feet feel cold. Low thermometer readings are indicative of low metabolism and low thyroid. Typically, a quarter or half grain of *Armour thyroid* raises temperatures back to a more normal 98.6° F. The key indicators are low body temperature and cold hands and feet, *and not blood tests*. All of my physician colleagues are currently treating the symptoms and not the lab reports. Welcome to 21st century medicine as it should have been practiced twenty years ago.

I treat low thyroid since it is known in the medical literature (Table Two) to increase one's chances of dying by about 33%. On the other hand, animals that hibernate can thrive on low thyroid since their energy factories or *mitochondria* work efficiently at *even* low levels of metabolic activity. Unfortunately, humans cannot unless they raise the efficiency of their mitochondria by consuming optimal amounts of strong antioxidants at every meal – the Lippman one pill/one meal protocol.

Please get your thyroid and testosterone on track in accordance with Tables One and Two if your expect to live much longer than the typical USA life expectancy of 74 years for men and 77 years for women. It works.

Table 1

Thresholds: **Male testosterone normal values and their deficiency thresholds accompanied by various symptoms[2]**

- **1100 to 1400** ng/dl total serum T = typical young male T range[1].

- **750 to 850** = optimal T range for men over forty that helps to reduce prostate cancer risk by 83%[8] and metabolic syndrome by 92%[9]. Also, the following problems of andropause are avoided at this optimal range:

- **432** = loss of libido and/or vigor[4], pale faced, lack of shiny eyes.

- **288** = depression[3], grumpiness[3], diabetes mellitus Type II[7], arterial stiffness[5], Alzheimer's[4], and approximately 8% thickening of the carotid arteries[6].

- **231** = erectile dysfunction[3], sarcopenia[10], arterial-vascular disease[1].

Notes: (a) Many men over 60 years of age are T deficient with values from 250 and 350 ng/dl total serum. Using T replacement therapy, raising 350 to 550 decreases chances of dying by 41%. Further elevating T in 200 point increments reduces chances of dying by 14% with each increment. (b) Men with proven coronary heart disease showed T values < 611.[1] (c) Sarcopenia: half of all people over the age of 70 cannot rise from a chair without the use of their hands[11]. T eliminates urinary incontinence in 6 days when combined with "stop/start" urinary exercises[12].

Table 2

Thresholds: Treatment with Armour® thyroid based on frequency of symptoms at various basal axillary temperatures according to:

98.6° F = normal basal axillary temperature in healthy individuals.

<97.4° F = tired and "on edge",[3] myxedema (swelling) of the ankles and lower legs.[2]

<97.0° F = fatigue and exhaustion (90%), asthma (85%), nausea (90%), allergic rhinitis and other allergies (80%), irregular menses (99%), palpitation (99%), poor concentration (95%).[1]

<96.4° F[1] = depression and "feeling lousy," brittle splitting nails, dry skin and hair and hair loss, sluggish thought processes, high cholesterol and triglycerides[1+3].

<95.8° = reduced libido and cold intolerance.[1]

Notes: The important heart hormone, T3 protects against arrhythmias. Low T3 and not high cholesterol is the strongest predictor of cardiac death. Men over 50 with low T3 have a 33% increased rate of death. Sub-clinical hypothyroidism means infarct. A minimum of 200 mg magnesium plus 150 mcg of T3 + T4 needed daily for a healthy heart. Half of 50 to 70 year old men have a bioavailable T3 level below the lowest level of healthy 20 to 40 year old men. Natural killer cells (NK) are the primary defense against cancer, and T3 increases NK cells. Minimum consumption of 12 mg daily of iodine and iodide essential, especially if thyroid size is irregular. References: Doctors Ron Rothenberg and Thierry Hertoghe, *International Hormone Society Meeting,* San Diego, CA, Sept. 2007.

Table 3

Thresholds: For those over 45, bio-identical progesterone (P) needed to alleviate the following deficiencies or systems

- 15 to 20 mg/d (about 28 ng/dl serum) for typical deficiencies [1]: Men may be puffy and red faced. Also, uterine fibroids, fibrocystic breasts, mild asthma, PMS, menstrual bleeding, osteoporosis, depression, water retention, decreased libido, sweets cravings, and excess fat deposition[8]. Furthermore, breast, uterine, ovarian, cervical, vaginal, and colon cancers[3].

- 50 to 100 mg/d typical deficiencies of men with BPH (benign prostate hypertrophy)[2], lower sperm count, depression, low libido, low DHEA, high serum estradiol, cardiovascular disease, hirsutism (excess hair), male pattern baldness, sleep problems and nightly nervous tension[16].

- 100 to 300 mg/d typical deficiencies in estrogen-dominant woman and sometimes in men[3]. DHEA increases up to 100% when 120 mg/d P applied[8]. Migraine headaches remedied[8]. Blood sugar normalized. Obesity prevented. Libido optimized. Natural anti-depressant and energizer[8]. Hard or enlarged prostate in about one third of all men[16].

- 300 mg/d typically needed to alleviate ADHD in adolescents and fibromyalgia[3].

- 300 to 400 mg/d (about 450 ng/dl serum) normal production of P during last trimester of pregnancy[8].

- 800 mg/d (400 mg 2X daily) for 4 months essential to maintain a healthy pregnancy in deficient women[3].

Notes: P inhibits 5-alpha reductase, and thus limits conversion of T to DHT which decreases hyperplasia induced by estradiol in men[5]. 100 mg P reduces estradiol by 30%[16]. P prevents post-menopausal bone loss[6]. Estradiol increases cancer cell growth; whereas supplementing with P stops this growth[7]. Adequate levels of P balance estradiol cell proliferation and may prevent up to 90% of all breast cancers. P decreased proliferation 400%[11]. P inhibits cancer due to p13 kinase/AKT pathway causing apoptosis of breast cancer cells[12]. 100 years ago, 1 of 94 women developed breast cancer; today, 1 of 8[3]. Pre-cancer cell changes are probably related to P deficiency[8]. Mild to moderate endometriosis remedied by P[8]. Fibrocystic lumps disappear after 2 to 4 months of P suppository use[3]. In post-menopausal women, extra P induces loss of facial hair and restoration of thinned scalp hair[8]. Both contraceptive pills and synthetic progestins or Provera inhibit natural production of P and lower DHEA levels[8]. P works best with magnesium 375 mg/d, Vitamin B6, and zinc 30 mg/d. P lowers LDL and raises HDL[9]. P is thermogenic and burns fat[3]. Insulin overproduced when P deficient[3]. Physiologic levels of both estradiol and P decrease foam cell formation[10]. P prevents reduces platelet aggregation and increases nitric oxide relaxing vascular endothelium[13]. P inhibits vascular cell adhesion molecules thereby decreasing endothelial inflammation[14]. P up-regulates nitric oxide synthase activity in vaginal tissue. Adequate female sexual response requires adequate levels of P [15]. Approx. 2 years before menopause, women stop ovulating and P production stops. P causes expectant mothers' radiant appearance[3]. P best taken before bedtime but without aldosterone supplements[16].

Table 4

Thresholds: DHEA serum values and deficiency thresholds accompanied by various symptoms:

200 to 610 mcg/dl reference range young adult men[1].

80 to 480 mcg/dl reference range young women[1].

280 mcg/dl women **or** 400 mcg/dl men, respectively, optimal values of DHEA[1]. Values exceeding these may indicate DHEA excess characterized by oily hair, skin, and acne.

94.5 to 100 mcg/dl threshold: increased arterial stiffness, intima-media thickness, impaired glucose tolerance, hyperglycemia, liver disease, diabetes. HbA1C inversely related to DHEA concentration.[2]

54.5 mcg/dl threshold: risk of dying increases by 64%[3].

33 to 39 mcg/dl threshold: Sparse or reduced area of pubic or armpit hair[1]. 2) Rheumatoid arthritis[4]. 3) Alzheimer's[4], 4) Depression[10] 5) Sexual dysfunction[9] 6) Abnormal brain MRI scan of grey matter. 7) increased cardiovascular and cancer mortalities[5,6].

Notes: Other problems associated with low serum DHEA include aggressive prostate cancer[5], aggressive cancers in women[6], increased BMI and hip circumference in young women[7], persistent acne in women[8], sexual dysfunction in women[9], depression in adolescents[10] and increase risk of cataract[11].

The Promise of the New Millennium: Replacement and Supplementation
What is normal to me and 2,000 board-certified anti-aging physicians worldwide are the hormonal test scores of healthy, young people in their twenties or perhaps in their thirties.

If these hormones become deficient as we age, think how that could adversely affect our health and lifespan. Consider carefully what replacement of deficient hormones would mean to our health and energy in our 60s, 70s, 80s and beyond. Some doubting friends of mine have exclaimed, "But it's not normal to replace them. Nature didn't intend our declining hormones and sagging bodies to be replaced or repaired!" I always retort, "Just because old-age debilitation is normal, doesn't mean we shouldn't try to do something about it. Isn't this what medicine in the 21st century should be focusing upon? Isn't this the promise of the new millennium?"

Of course, when attempting to return to normal from a state of hormone deficiencies, I should first define what "normal" means. Normal to me means the level of my hormones when I was in my thirties; however many other American anti-aging physicians define "normal" as the level one had in one's twenties. I choose a different level since I refuse the libido of a 20 year old. This is my personal choice, but to each their own. Whatever you decide, please note that the only way to safely and responsibly replace hormones is to seek the help of a *knowledgeable* anti-aging physician. They understand that many of our hormones decline during aging. By careful testing with blood, urine, and saliva samples, they can identify hormone deficiencies and implement replacement therapy which can result in a concrete promise of health and longevity in the third millennium. These specialists understand that the size and weight of our bodies has not decreased since our twenties, and therefore, why should we settle for lower hormone amounts that incorrectly support our current body masses? We definitely need the same amount of hormones like we had back in our thirties, and in fact some people with exaggerated libidos sincerely desire to return to their sex hormone levels at age 20! However, I am perfectly satisfied with my sex hormone testosterone-level at age 35. This level gives me the correct amount of libido while balancing my intellectual and emotional needs--but to each his or her own. In any case, I definitely want to avoid becoming hormonally challenged.

What does "normal" really mean to medical professionals? Should normal be defined as a decline in our mental and muscular abilities as we age? No way. Strangely, *"normal" to many medical practitioners has been based on the blood and urine test-scores of sick patients*. These standards are ill-conceived and incorrect for me and my love ones. We demand the hormone levels of healthy people in their twenties and thirties, and we are more than willing to pay for that privilege outside of regular HMO and Medicare health plans that refuse anti-aging medicine.

Despite what you may have been led to believe, the government is not willing to extend your lifespan and continue paying you Social Security benefits. You must do this on your own – a form of self-empowerment. You decide on your desired level of health and vitality, and avoid becoming hormonally challenged. Hopefully you will make a decision to empower yourself during the coming revolution of anti-aging medicine.

Friends of mine read the preceding paragraphs and asked me point blank what to ask their current physician about anti-aging medicine. I replied that most physicians remain unaware about anti-aging medicine, especially hormones, anti-cross linkers, and free radicals, since these subjects are not currently being taught by medical schools. Again, aging is a natural process, and medical schools only teach disease. However, I believe that anti-aging medicine truly is the cutting-edge medicine of the future. Only those health care professionals who have the edge and take *advanced* courses in hormones and anti-aging medicine will help you. In this regard, in the US over 2,000 physicians are board-certified in anti-aging medicine with The American Academy of Anti-Aging Medicine. Other American physicians are not board certified, but they may well be very knowledgeable in the field. These physicians often acquired their advanced knowledge by completing AMA courses where they accumulated points from The Accreditation Council for Continuing Medical Education, accessible at www.meccine.com.

From a practical point of view, knowledgeable anti-aging

physicians can be sourced by phoning the nearest "compounding pharmacy" in the city where you live. Compounding pharmacies are specialty pharmacies that make *custom* formulations of prescription products such as bio-identical hormones. Your local compounder will know all physicians in your area who are skilled at anti-aging medicine and use compounders to custom tailor various hormones to the *exact* needs of an individual patient. For example, instead of ordering an off-the-shelf progesterone cream available only 100 or 200 mg doses, a compounding pharmacist can custom fill your order for 130 mg or any other dose prescribed by your physician. Freedom to customize pharmaceutical products is yet another milestone of 21st century anti-aging medicine which should be enjoyed and appreciated by all those who value individual freedom.

In summary, what is normal to me and thousands of knowledgeable anti-aging physicians worldwide are the hormonal test scores of healthy, young people in their twenties or perhaps in their thirties (my choice) and not values based on the sick and elderly. Your choice. This entire scenario reminds me of what my mother as an R.N. told me of her medical experiences in the 40's and 50's. She worked closely with a Dr. Furnish, and the two of them encouraged patients to take vitamin supplements. Other doctors at that time would usually chuckle and say that vitamin supplements were a waste of money or even harmful. You decide.

I have a question for all Doubting Thomases of anti-aging therapy: Would you like to live sixty Frank Sinatra years or one hundred Spiro Agnew years? I always answer that my loved ones and I want to live 150 Sinatra years and let the aging nay-Sayers enjoy premature aging and their strollers, bingo, and shuffleboard. Let us move forward with all activities that would improve the health and the quality of our senior years. These activities would include routine comprehensive lab tests of our essential hormones to determine if any are too high or too low. I highly recommend the "Age Management Panel™" testing as provided by Meridian Valley Laboratory in Renton, Washington. (See www.meridianvalleylab.com for requisition of test forms.) Another favorite by the same lab is their Comprehensive Plus Hormone Profile with HGH. Anyone can order these tests without prescription or medical help, but the results may be difficult to interpret without the assistance of a knowledgeable anti-aging physician or other hormone expert. However, Meridian Valley's on site hormone expert will personally discuss your lab results with you free of charge, but your understanding of the results will be limited without knowledgeable physician help. Believe me, hormones as well as rocket science and nuclear physics are all very tough to understand.

Unlike previous chapters, I cannot make many personal recommendations as to what hormones you should be taking since such suggestions must be based upon complete lab testing, especially *24-hour urine tests*. These testing methods reveal many hormones and their byproducts or metabolites not usually determined by blood and saliva testing methods. This means collecting your total urine output during a period of 24 hours and mailing in two samples of your combined urine sample to a specialty lab. For example, Meridian Valley Labs determines two critical hormone metabolites, the carcinogens, *4 and 16 alpha hydroxyestrones*. Science classifies them as *genotoxic* which means they will alter your genes such as DNA. If you test for them, and they appear in your lab results, your physician might help you to eliminate them through simple therapeutic treatment. In other words, *testing is essential*, and then and only then can your therapy begin. Hormones are a complex subject, and one must rely upon truly knowledgeable physicians for help. I apologize for not having found a simpler way. I personally test myself quarterly and regularly apply progesterone and testosterone creams and consume a little thyroid hormone. They work, trust me.

Recommendations

- If you can afford 310 dollars, get tested with a comprehensive 24 hour urine panel to achieved better balance of your hormones and avoid many of the ravages of aging.

Golden Keys to Longevity #5

- *Longevity and good health are mortally dependent upon a balanced symphony of hormones such as progesterone, aldosterone, cortisone, human growth hormone, testosterone, the estrogens, and thyroid hormone.*

- *Hormones are the rate-limiting step that deficiencies prevent us from living to at least our nineties.*

References to Table 1

1. Notes: Ron Rothenburg MD, International Hormone Society Meeting, Las Vegas, NV, Feb. 2008.
2. Thresholds: Zitzmann, M, Faber S, Nieschlag E, Association of specific symptoms and metabolic risks with serum testosterone in older men. J Clin. Endocrinol. Metab. 2006 Nov, 91(11), pp. 4335-43. Muller M, et al, J Clin Endocrinol Metab. 2005 Aug 90(8), p.4979. Mortality thresholds: Mohr BA, Clin Endocrinol (Oxf.) 2005 Jan, 62(1), pp. 64-73.
3. Depression and ED: Makhlouf AA, Neiderberger C, Hypogonadism is associated with overt depression symptoms in men with erectile dysfunction. Int. J. Impot. Res. 2007 Aug. 16.
4. Alzheimer's: Moffat SD, Zonderman AB, Metter EJ, Kawas C, Blackman MR, Harman SM, Resnick SM, Free testosterone and risk for Alzheimer disease in older men, Neurology, 2004 Jan 27, 62(2) pp.188-93.
5. Arterial stiffness: Fukui M, Ose H, Kitagawa Y, Yamazaki M, Hasegawa G, Yoshikawa T, Nakamura N, Relationship between low serum endogenous androgen concentrations and arterial stiffness in men with Type 2 diabetes mellitus. Metabolism 2007 Sept. 56(9), pp. 1167-73.
6. Carotid thickening: Mäkinen J, Huhtaniemi I, Raitakari OT, Increased carotid atherosclerosis in andropausal middle-aged men. J Am Coll. Cardiol. 2005, 45(10), pp. 1603-8.
7. Type II diabetes: Ding EL, Song Y, Malik VS, Liu S, Sex differences of endogenous sex hormones and risk of type 2 diabetes, JAMA 2006 Mar 295(11), pp. 1288-99, Harvard Medical School, Boston
8. Prostate: Severi G, Cancer Epidemiol. Biomarkers Prev, 2006, 15(1), pp. 86-91.

9. Muller M et al, J Clin Endocrinol Metab, 2005 Aug ,90(8), p. 4979.

10. Sarcopenia: Iannuzzi-Sucich M, Prestwood KM, Kenny AM, Prevalence of carcopenia and skeletal muscle mass in healthy, older men and women, J Geront. A Biol Sci Med Sci, 2002 Dec 57(12), pp. 772-777. Univ. Of Connecticut.

11. Sarcopenia: Robert Willix, MD, 2007 Nov, Age Management Meeting, Red Rock, Nevada.

12. Incontinence: Michael E. Platt, 2007, *Miracle of Bio-Identical Hormones,* Clancy Lane Pub., Rancho Mirage, CA.

References to Table 2

Misc. references:
1. ACAM or Amer. College Advancement of Med. Meeting, Chicago, Ill, March 2007.

2. Alan R. Gaby MD, Alternative Med. Review, 2004 vol. 9 (2), pp. 157-179.

3. Neal Rouzier MD, *How to Achieve Health Aging,* 2007, World Link Publ, pp.165-173.

References to Table 3:

1. John R. Lee Newsletter, March 1999, p. 7.

2. Ibid Feb. 1999, p. 7.

3. Platt, Michael E., 2007, *Miracle of Bio-Identical Hormones,* Clancy Lane Publishing, Rancho Mirage, CA.

4. John R. Lee Newsletter, March 1999, p. 2.

5. Ibid Jan. 1999, p. 3.

6. Leonetti, H. B. et al., Obstetrics & Gynecology, Vol. 94(2), pp. 225-228.

7. Formby, B. and Wiley, T.S., John R. Lee Newsletter, June 1998, p. 3.

8. Shealy, C. Norman, 1999, *Natural Progesterone Cream,* Keats Pub., Los Angeles, CA.

9. 1989, Obstet. Gyn., Vol. 73, pp. 606-611.

10. 1999, Circulation, Dec 7, Vol. 100, pp. 2319-2325.
11. 1995, Fertility Sterility, Vol. 63, pp. 785-791.
12. 2002, Eur. J. Cancer Prev., Oct, Vol. 11(5), pp. 481-488.
13. 1992, Eur. J. Pharmacol. Vol. 201, pp. 163-167.
14. 2001 Feb, Arterioscler. Thromb. Vasc. Vol. 21(2), pp. 243-249.
15. 1999, Neurobiology of Sexual Behavior, Vol. 9, pp. 751-758.
16. Hertoghe, Thierry, 2006, *The Hormone Handbook*, Int. Med. Pub., Surrey, UK.

References to Table 4

1. International Hormone Society Meeting, Preventative and Regenerative Medicine, Thierry Hertoghe, MD, 2008 Oct 23-26, pp.362-373, and "*The Hormone Handbook*" 2006, Int. Medical Pub., Surry, UK, pp. 293 to 295.
2. Recent Prog. Med. 1989, 80 (1) pp. 4-8. and Am. J. Physiol. Endocrinol. Metab., 2006 Feb, 290(2) pp. E234-242.
3. Taiwanese Ann. Epidemiol. 2006 Jul, 16(7) pp. 510515.
4. Ann N Y Acad. Sci. 2006 Jun, 1069, pp. 223-235. and Sunderland T et al, 1989, Lancet, 2 p. 570.
5. Cancer Epidemiol Biomarkers Prev. 2006 Jan, 15(1) pp. 86-91.
6. J Gerontol A Biol Sci Med Sci 2006 Sept, 61(9) pp. 957-962.
7. Saudi Med J 2003 Aug 24(8) pp. 837-841.
8. Arch Dematol 2005 Mar 141(3) pp. 333-338.
9. J Sex Martal Ther. 2002, Suppl. 1 pp. 165-173.
10. Psychol Med 2003 May 33(4) pp. 601-610.
11. Ann Epidemiol 2003 Oct 13(9) pp 638-644.

Chapter 6
Ban Free Radicals!

Optimizing Antioxidants that Prevent Free-Radical Damage
"If you suppress free radicals, you suppress programmed cell death."
Rudolph Salganik, MD, Ph.D., D. Sc.

When I began my study of free radicals, I was a lone voice in the wilderness. Fate had cast me as a wolf howling on a lonely prairie for lost companions. I was obsessed by the work of Professor Denham Harman who proved that *strong* antioxidants increased mean lifespan in mice by fifty percent. But I did not know where his research could take me and what to do upon arrival. I toyed with strategies *to measure* the aging process. If only I could use my measurement skills, the payoff for slowing aging could be significant. My loved ones and mankind would benefit. But the question remained how to achieve measurement. I attended many medical meetings in the hopes of acquiring a handle on how to proceed. Much to my horror I discovered that other doctors were uninterested in measuring anything except disease. Worse were the prevailing attitudes of the pop culture which encouraged gobbling mega-doses of vitamins without consideration of the consequences. This monochromatic view was wrong, and I rode forth to correct the world in spite of prevailing notions, illusions, and prejudices.

I worked and studied alone with the vexing problems of measurement until one day I read that Professor Harman held regular scientific meetings with his group called "AGE" (American Aging Association). Then I realized that aging could at least be studied and that AGE scientists such as Dr. Ward Dean shared my interests. I hoped to find fellow scientists who appreciated my methods in spite of being ignored by the public. I became motivated since future discoveries would benefit everyone, especially my family.

In this chapter, I summarize some of my work since it remains unmistakably a complex subject. In fact because of its complexity, it is rather like writing one of those "How to for Dummies" books on nuclear physics or rocket science – impossible tasks to say the least. Therefore, please bear with me, and I will endeavor to advance my best efforts in simplifying the complicated and not complicating the simple.

This chapter explains my revolutionary probes invented by me for special measurement of free radicals in human cells. With the help of these probes and other scientific instruments, I detailed how free radicals and other related *active oxygens* such as ozone and carbon monoxide can be avoided for better health and longevity.

Apparently, effective remedies for retarding aging should use truly STRONG antioxidants and free-radical scavengers – not weak ones such as Vitamins C and E that are promoted ad nauseam in the US pop culture.

This chapter is worth reading since its research paved the way to my nomination for the Nobel Prize in Medicine. Therefore, please have patience.

Background to my Nomination
A quest to slow Father Time in spite of Mother Nature's many roadblocks.

Ever since the US Patent Office accepted my breakthrough patent entitled, "*Methods for Retarding Aging*," I lectured tirelessly in a quest to slow Father Time in spite of Mother Nature's many roadblocks. At these lectures, scientists and physicians would applaud me and repeatedly exclaim that I should receive the Nobel Prize in Medicine for my many innovations. I felt undeserving. I really only wanted to help people. Becoming a Nobel laureate meant rising to the top of my profession, a heady thought. But after hearing their praises for the umpteenth time, I disregarded their accolades and renewed my focus on research and my family's needs. My family required emotional and economic support, and these needs were uppermost in my mind. Praise could wait.

Then one sunny day, a letter arrived with a return address from the Nobel Prize Committee. I tore it open with excitement and found a list of prominent scientists who had forwarded my name. I was formally nominated, and the news thrilled me and my loved ones. My long-sought scientific reputation was finally confirmed and honored. In the deadly business of defeating aging, I could not hope for more. Years of lecturing and research had finally scored their mark. Bravo for the Nobel Prize Committee.

The Scourge of Free Radicals
Active oxygens such as ozone slowly and insidiously destroy our skin and arteries in a decades-long hardening and cracking process. Although this is only one aspect of the aging process, we can do something to remedy it.

My father and grandfather were very large building contractors, and they instilled in me a desire to discover why things work and if they did not, how one might remedy the situation. This established my male bonding ritual with them. I became the student asking questions. One cold morning I remember my father led me into a blackened, burnt-out building. It had suffered smoke damage, and I asked him how to fix the lingering smell of burnt wood. He suggested tenting the building and flooding it with ozone gas for three days.

In later years I likened this blackened, burnt-out building to what happens in our bodies with aging. During aging our bodies suffer a type of smoke damage since we live in a world rich with active oxygens. In fact, twenty percent of the air we breathe is composed of *oxygen*. If you doubt this statement, observe the rubber wind-shield wipers on your car. After many months of exposure to active oxygens in the air, this rubber becomes brittle and cracks and needs replacement. Oxygen surrounds us daily and supports our metabolism but at the same time can be deleterious to our health. Oxygen is a double-edged sword.

However, just as buildings can be fixed, likewise with damage to our bodies caused by aging. These methods may involve ozone, but even more effective is the use of truly *strong* antioxidants that prevent unwanted oxidations. Allow me to introduce a simplified explanation as follows.

My father's burned-out building suffered smoke damage from fire and the toxin, *carbon monoxide, or* CO, while during aging, similar active oxygens damage our bodies. The building's CO damage can be reversed by tenting it over and flooding it with ozone or O3 gas for three days. The same mitigating process may be used in our aging bodies by treatment with ozone, or better still with *strong* antioxidants.

Carbon monoxide caused a pungent smell in the burned-out building from incomplete carbon combustion, a process which adds only *one* oxygen atom to it. On the other hand, if it underwent complete combustion, adding a second oxygen would convert it to CO2 or *carbon dioxide,* an odorless gas. Carbon monoxide and burnt wood have pungent-sweet smells neutralized with ozone.

A further example reveals itself in the cracking of car tires in ozone-rich cities like Los Angeles and Mexico City. The O3 reacts with rubber side-walls and damages them. Tires become cracked and hardened and must be periodically replaced. Automobile rubber is composed of unsaturated chemical bonds that will readily bond to ozone. When this occurs, rubber loses its *structural integrity*. In the human body we call these bonding chemicals "polyunsaturated fatty acids," and a very similar process happens in the body over many years. Active oxygens such as ozone insidiously destroy our skin and arteries in a decades-long hardening and cracking process. Although only one aspect of the aging process, we can do something to remedy it as in the case of the burned-out building. My lifelong quest sought to discover why active oxygens may adversely affect living organisms, especially humans.

Regarding another practical example of active oxygens, I would like to share a patient case history from the files of my friend and associate, Ward Dean, MD. Dr. Dean's patient, Mr. Barkley, had suffered for many years from an unspecified variety of symptoms that other physicians were unable to identify with a concrete diagnosis. Dr. Dean suggested several cleansing therapies. Mr. B wondered if the drinking of ozone-treated water combined with iodine plus antioxidants would work.

Dr. Dean answered that Mr. B asked a very good question to which he did not have a definitive answer, and he did not know if anyone else did either. Combining intravenous hydrogen peroxide with ozone gas as well as photo-luminescent irradiation of blood would perhaps induce the body to produce its own higher levels of antioxidants. However, if Mr. B wished to increase his antioxidants, then Dr. Dean suggested switching to *N-acetyl-cysteine* and *l-glutathione*. Furthermore, Dr. Dean recommended this book written by his good friend, namely me, that addresses some of these concerns such as optimizing with antioxidant therapy. In conclusion, Dr. Dean said that the bottom line seems to be that these two therapies do not counteract each other but may work in a complementary fashion.

I replied that based on my research, I fully concur with Dr. Dean. Drinking ozonated water becomes neutralized in the stomach, and it provides a mild anti-bacterial effect similar to chlorinated water or hot chili-peppers. The ozone does not reach the blood stream in significant quantities. On the other hand, iodine and strong antioxidants such as N-acetyl cysteine and l-glutathione are easily absorbed through the stomach lining into the blood stream and positively impact all organs and tissues.

As mentioned earlier, I became interested in active oxygens called *nitroso* compounds responsible for the carcinogens (cancer causing agents) in fried bacon and other processed meats. This work led to the discovery that many organic substances containing sulphur could destroy nitroso carcinogens and other active oxygens. In 1977, I observed that organic sulfurs could be rapidly *measured* in tiny amounts using my special chemical marking system. These unique chemical markers, or *probes,* could rapidly identify and quantify organic sulfurs, their poisonous cousins, nitroso compounds, and other active oxygens. My probes gave off light in varying intensities and in proportion to various oxidants and antioxidants.

This light is called *chemiluminescense* (chemically-induced *cold light*), since it requires a chemical reaction much like the *emergency light-sticks* used by motorists. Fireflies and glow worms provide everyday examples of this cold light which biologist even have labeled as *bioluminescence* (biologically-induced *cold light*).

During the 1973 Middle-East war, Israeli pilots saw underwater lights moving across the Red Sea. They believed that the lights originated from Egyptian frogmen and proceeded to bomb them. In actual fact, the lights emanated from bioluminescent bacteria on the eyelids of rare Red Sea fish. These fish blinked their eyelids to attract their mates using this unique form of symbioses. Young ladies paint their eyelids for the same reason!

For a long time scientists believed that the free-radical processes in test tubes acted similar to those in the cells of mammals. But I became convinced that this oversimplified a complex process. Obviously, a living organism such as a mouse or a human being is much more chemically complicated. But the question remained: how to move from a test tube to an experimental model of a living organism?

My specially synthesized chemiluminescent probes penetrated locations within rat and human cells. More specifically they probed the mitochondria of the cells where poisonous free-radicals and active oxygens are generated. Consequently, these probes monitored and measured the normal occurrence of free radicals, peroxides, active oxygens, and cell-membrane damages. Anti-aging nutrients were introduced and their efficiencies compared, evaluated, and even optimized. This led to the development of different anti-aging mixtures and an optimal lowering of poisonous cell oxidations.

Revolutionary Measurement of Free Radicals inside Human Cells
My cold-light probes captured the production of the superoxide radical in full-flow detail.

I put on my thinking cap and imagined how to test and even *measure* free radicals in living systems. I knew that if I could accomplish this feat, everyone would benefit from limiting free radicals cascading throughout the body like a waterfall of shooting stars. Chemical probes would achieve this goal. Every day I hastened to my lab, and the excitement of achieving the near impossible became my motivator.

I imagined a solution involving the creation of these special chemiluminescent (*cold light*) *probes.* I synthesized them by combining a known chemiluminescent substance, *luminol* with another chemical entity known for easy entry through cell membranes.

What did I discover with my probes? In 1979 the first experiments revealed that the burning of oxygen in the cells' energy factories was not 100% efficient. This fact mirrored the known efficiency of large electric motors where 97% of their electrical energy converts into motion and 3% becomes wasted as heat. Similarly, the burning of oxygen in the mitochondria of humans is only 94 to 98% efficient and 2 to 6% becomes wasted. Low efficiency means lower than normal body temperature and hypothyroidism – the later known to shorten lifespan up to 33%.

This is my original discovery. The wasted oxygen piqued my interest since it consisted of free radicals and peroxides known to be extremely dangerous to living systems. In bacteria only approximately 83% of oxygen efficiently converts itself. No one in the scientific community had these exact efficiency figures. Subsequently, in 1979 and in later years this research led to my other unique discoveries such as:

- Understanding the molecular mechanisms governing the mitochondria's energy factories.
- Raising mitochondrial efficiency to the 97% upper limit in order to avoid hypothyroidism.
- Viewing the generation of free radicals cascading from those energy factories and envisioning damage.
- Challenging the cascading free radicals with free-radical scavengers.
- Optimizing suspected scavengers.
- Employing other types of chemiluminescent probes.
- Confirming that free radicals are some of the most poisonous chemicals on the planet and greatly contribute to human illness and aging.
- Confirming that free radicals are generated in estrogen dominant people who have excessive 4-hydroxyestrogens –

the one and only proven cause of ovarian cancer. (Pharmacotherapy, 2003, 23(2), pp. 165-172.)

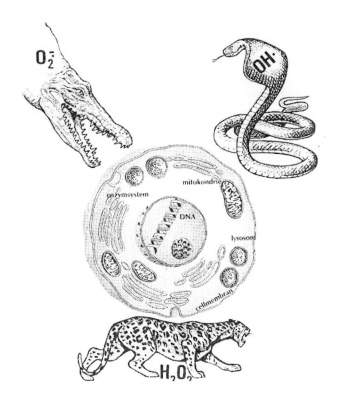

Figure One. A simple human cell with structures: mitochondria (the cell's energy factories); lysosomes (the cell's garbage dump); and the cell nucleus (the cell's genes or DNA). The cell is bombarded continually 24/7 by free radicals and other active oxygens. I probed these structures to determine free-radical activity and likely counter measures.

America's leading gerontology journals first published my unique discoveries in *Experimental Gerontology,* 1980, 15, pages 339-351, and *Journal of Gerontology*, 1981, vol. 36, No.5, pages 550-557. I remember appearing many times in New York City in the early 80s at

AGE meetings hosted by Professor Denham Harman. I lectured extensively on my discoveries and their significance to anti-aging research. At subsequent AGE meetings, I presented further findings from my unique research. My Swedish professors and other scientists, such as my newfound friend Ward Dean, MD, were convinced that my research was revolutionary. However, few grants were awarded since the medical world lacked interest in anti-aging research. With this in mind, research involving diseases and disease processes became my priority in order to secure grant money. Some scientists such as Professor Harman, Dr. Linus Pauling, Dr. Garry Gordon, and Dr. Ward Dean, with strong backgrounds in both chemistry and medicine, understood my accomplishment. It would take another ten to twenty years for the medical world to grudgingly acknowledge the critical role of free radicals in disease and in the aging process.

The Testing Stage and Resulting Benefits
Typically weak antioxidants like Vitamins C and E have little effect upon free radicals and the aging process, as compared with strong antioxidants, BHT, BHA, NDGA, DMSA, and ethoxyquin.

During late 1979, I returned to my lab and began to consider the practical applications of my probe research. I loved scientific theory, but since I am a practical person like my father and grandfather, I wanted to see concrete results. I began to wonder how this research could benefit my own health, and offer greater longevity to my loved ones and humanity in general. I drew up lists of chemical substances that were either known or suspected to neutralize free radicals and extend life. The most obvious substances were those researched by Professor Denham Harman, namely *BHT* and *BHA*. Prof. Harman had previously proven that these substances could increase the average lifespan of mice by at least 50% and reduced incidence of stomach cancer in American soldiers. A third substance, *ethoxyquin* from Monsanto, had successfully extended egg-laying lifespan in commercial chickens by 30-40%. This powerful antioxidant was sold to commercial poultry farms during the 60s. All these strong antioxidants raised mitochondrial efficiency. See Figure Two. The results are described in Appendix B.

Santoquin˙ Antioxidant
(ethoxyquin)
can it actually slow the process
of aging?

Figure Two. Monsanto Chemical Co. sold a powerful free radical scavenger, Ethoxyquin to commercial poultry farmers who increased chicken lifespan and egg laying up to 41%.

Finding the Best Antioxidants and Using Them Correctly
Others had tried and arrived at solutions that did not pan out.

I knew that elimination of cellular garbage was an important goal for the health of humanity during aging. But an even more important goal was the comparison of nutrients that would render harmless free radicals in humans. I wanted to save humanity from the toxic indignities of the relentless assault of cascading free radicals, especially their cancer, artery, and skin hardening effects. Others had tried and arrived at solutions that did not pan out. Their solutions involved *mega dosing* with large handfuls of antioxidants in the hopes that free radicals would all become quenched (inactivated) and cell metabolism became more efficient and optimized.

But unfortunately, Professor Denham Harman proved them all wrong in the early 80's. Mega dosing does not work. In fact, it *increases* the rate of aging due to the pro-oxidant effects of high dose antioxidants. I too had my problems in my lab. While I identified effective and ineffective antioxidants, I could not optimize dosage levels due to experimental difficulties. Therefore, all dosage recommendations remain only "good" estimates of effective destruction of free radicals. But the benefits of these estimates appear significant in slowing *this* aspect of the aging.

Nutrients that Protect Human Brain Cells
My one pill/one meal regimen results in reduced stickiness of every cell in the body. Your future health and longevity rests upon this basic fact.

I wanted to help aging humanity in other ways than just cosmetic treatment of skin. I sincerely wanted to protect humanity from the scourge of damaged brain cells during aging. Brain cells remain *more* important to me and my loved ones than a little skin discoloration and a trip to Neiman Marcus for their latest beauty tip. Basic knowledge of brain cell chemistry, especially free-radical and hormone chemistry, became an important research goal. To this end I found a supply of volunteers who would donate samples of their brain cells. This sourcing was difficult to obtain in spite of the fact that many people daily sacrifice millions of brain cells to aging and to over-consumption of alcohol. Organ and cell donations remain difficult to find in the case of medical research. Suffice it to say, I received needed cells for completion of my research, and humanity has benefited.

I impregnated human brain cells and tested them with a special probe. Results showed that BHT, ACF 228, RNA, Vitamin E, testosterone, and hydrocortisone protected brain-cell lysosomes from superoxide free radicals. *This was my special discovery.* Iron seems to promote free radical activity, as well as copper and choline which showed some negative effects. Copper seems beneficial in a cell's energy factories, or mitochondria, *but* detrimental in a cell's waste disposal bags (lysosomes).

Therefore, I conclude that only really *powerful* antioxidants and free radical scavengers effectively limit free-radical cascading in the human brain and further optimized metabolism. These results were unsurprising since they correlate with experiments conducted by others, namely Drs. Harman, Al Tappel, and Dean. Secondly, I discovered that consuming these supplements with every meal sustained high blood levels during any 24-hour period. My innovation. Thirdly, from these results I proposed the one pill/one meal regimen described earlier. My one pill/one meal regimen (minimum 250 mg) of truly strong antioxidants or nutrients remains a simple means to protect the body from free radical damage and aging. I have followed this one pill/one meal regimen since 1979 and the benefits have been worthwhile. My biological age is at least 15 to 20 years younger than my chronological age, and I remain disease free and in good health due to my multifaceted anti-aging regimen. For example, at age 63 my blood pressure measures a typical teenage level of 120 over 60.

I believe that consuming one pill with every meal is a slam-dunk step for everyone who desires slowed aging. I and my fellow scientists carry with us small aluminum-foil envelopes which contain multiple-meal supplies of strong antioxidants. Before every meal, I swallow one pill or capsule with water. If I measure the back of my hand on a special near-infrared instrument invented by me, I can monitor the absorption of this single pill or capsule into the blood stream approximately 45 minutes after taking it on an empty stomach. This allows monitoring its protective action during many hours. But please remember that consuming *mega* doses of nutrients may *accelerate* our rate of aging and cause metabolic imbalance.

Beware of mega-dose advertising claims. These claims may sound convincing, but they have not been monitored *pharmacokinetically* (*time-course study*) as my special *near*-infrared spectroscopy allows. These advertisers have not gone to the trouble and expense of discovering how various anti-aging substances really work in humans and at what optimal dosage levels.

Please consider the sobering fact that the marketing hype of the past has not yielded positive anti-aging results.

Another more long-term method of monitoring strong antioxidants employs a standard blood test taken before starting the one pill/one meal regimen. One may ask a doctor to order a *blood sedimentation* or "sed" test. After one or two months on the regimen, try testing one's sed rate again, and *one will discover that sed values have decreased dramatically to teenage levels.* For example, my older patients often begin with sed values over 25 and after two months of my regimen, their sed values decline to under 5. Note that the sed test determines how *sticky* one's red blood cells have become. In other words, if very sticky, red blood cells readily adhere to one another and rapidly sedimentise (clump together) in a test tube, and the sed rate becomes greater than 25. On the other hand, if they lack stickiness, red blood cells remain intact. They have not clumped together. Important: *red blood cells are health indicators of every cell in your body.* Thus, my one pill/one meal regimen results in reduced stickiness of *every cell in the body.* Everyone's health and longevity rests upon this basic fact.

Furthermore, some cells are the critical, *non-replicating cells of the heart, brain, and central nervous system.* If we lose too many of them, an organ dies and we die. Trust me. This key to longevity has often been ignored during the last twenty-five years. Also, this reflects the strongest direct proof of my regimen's benefits. These benefits of healthier, non-sticky cells throughout my body mean that I have more physical and mental energy than people decades younger than me. My sister, Cheryl often has commented that I have three times the energy of her friends in my age group, and guess what; energy is a function of mitochondria. Her friends who knew me more than 40 years ago usually exclaim that I look the same now as I did way back then. I most definitely have not discovered the fountain of youth, but I have stumbled upon several keys for improved health during my thirty years of research. You too can enjoy the wonderful longevity key of the one pill/one meal regimen.

Furthermore, we can strengthen and even optimize our defense systems by consuming extra quantities of strong antioxidants, membrane stabilizers, and hormones than our current diet allows. These will positively impact our rate of aging and susceptibility to the diseases and impairments often associated with aging, e.g., cancer, atherosclerosis, senility, memory loss, hypothyroidism, and declining sexual appetite.

The Scientific Explanation

Free Radicals' Role in Cancerous Estrogen Hormones

This book's introduction promised an indisputable connection between free radicals and hormones. This connection is explored in the renowned journal, Pharmacotherapy, 2003, 23(2), page 168. Estrogens related to *4-hydroxyestradiol* are the only known cause of ovarian cancer. 4-hydroxyestradiol is changed by enzymes (*peroxidases*) to free radicals, especially superoxide, which in turn causes DNA damage and cancer. As mentioned in the previous hormone chapters, blockers such as DIM, Arimidex, estriol, and 2-methoxyestradiol will prevent these cancers. Thus, hormones and free radicals are linked to one another in causing some of the diseases of aging, namely cancer and DNA damage. Ovarian as well as prostate and breast cancer can be prevented by consuming these blockers.

Pulling It All Together
Your chronological age will begin to diverge from your biological age.

To obtain that goal, one needs to commit to a 20-minute daily anti-aging regimen. This regimen would at *the very least* include 250 mg of a *strong* antioxidant or free-radical scavenger with every meal, daily consumption of anti-cross-linkers such as l-carnosine 250 mg, and aminoguanidine, 150 mg, and lastly, hormone replacement therapy, namely 75 mg daily DIM, 100 mcg (micrograms) daily estriol, or 200 mcg weekly Arimidex. Even this bare-bones daily practice will pay enormous dividends towards better health and slowed aging in the years to come. This is my promise to all readers of this book. Try this regimen and see if you do not feel healthier and happier, and your chronological age will begin to *diverge* from your biological age. Empower yourself. You only live once. Make this one go around more exciting and energetic – mitochondrial energetic.

Golden keys to longevity #6

- *Use moderate doses of strong antioxidants with every meal to prevent skin and organ free-radical damage during aging. Use anti-cancer hormone blockers to prevent free radicals in estrogen dominant people. Avoid mega doses of all nutrients to prevent pro-oxidation, mitochondrial inefficiency, and accelerated aging. An essential key to longevity is preserving the non-replicating cells of the heart, brain, and central nervous system with the 24/7 application of my special one pill/one meal regimen.*

Recommendations

- Consume the following blockers: 75 mg daily DIM, 100 mcg daily estriol, or 100 mcg twice weekly Arimidex.
- Also take *at least* 250 mg of any one or several of the following with each meal: Polyphenols, grape-seed extract, Pycnogenol, coenzyme Q10, BHT, BHA, ACF 228, Trolox C, l-methionine, l-cysteine (or N-acetyl cysteine), or l-glutathione.

Chapter 7
Supercharge Your Brain

Is Your Brain Receiving the Right Nutrients?

Recently a seventy year old man was the oldest one to climb mount Olympus. Unfortunately, he was overheard asking, 'What am I up here for"? Jay Leno

What Happens to an Aging Brain?
Three times she failed to respond to my simple questions. Low thyroid hormone had shifted her brain into a temporary mental fog.

Let us not pretend. Despite millions of dollars spent on brain research, the brain contains many unknowns. For example, we do not know why we sleep or what really causes Parkinson's and Alzheimer's. The first scientist to answer these riddles will no doubt receive numerous Nobel Prizes and the gratitude of humanity. In regards to aging, all we really know are some basic observations as to how the brain changes *physically and mentally during aging.*

Physically, it decreases from an average weight of 1,500 grams in a young adult to less than 1,000 grams in old age. A brain that has substantially decreased in size becomes highly forgetful, unable to memorize new information, and cannot react quickly to external stimuli. In fact, shrinkage and loss of function with age negatively impacts all organs in the body which corresponds to an accumulation of free-radical byproducts seen in the skin and elsewhere as wrinkles and age spots.

Mentally, scientists now know something about Parkinson's disease. At the cellular level Parkinson's victims lack *dopamine*, but after administering a close relative called *l-dopa* for only a year, it stops working and neuron deterioration continues. This causes irreversible damage to the brain and prevents it from sending electrical signals, and thus cognitive decline ensues. The body naturally produces l-dopa's cousin, a natural amino acid called *l-methionine*, which I consume daily 300 mg plus 50 mg Vitamin B-6, and I wash it down with grapefruit or pomegranate juice. The long term effects of these nutrients remain unknown, but allow me to inject that I have followed this therapy since 1979. Parkinson's disease remains a great mystery. Further research revelations await many more years of basic research. Anyone who says different is kidding himself and others.

In the case of Alzheimer's, the outlook is much brighter. Alzheimer's was first recognized by Dr. Alois Alzheimer in 1901 when he surprised colleagues by observing that patients had lost their identities and became confused and vegetative due to the accumulation of *sticky plaques* and *tangles* in their brains. These sticky plaques appeared under a microscope as crusty brown clumps which blocked communication between nerve cells; while the tangles highlighted themselves as weedy, menacing strands of rope growing wildly inside nerve cells.

According to two recent studies, cognitive abilities and underlying plaque improve when patients are given Enbrel®.

The current research focus of Big Pharma often aims at alleviating Alzheimer's *symptoms* and not curing the underlying disease. A great pity. My own research interest has always explored underlying hormonal, cross-linking, and free-radical *causes* of diseases and not just alleviating symptoms. To this end, I know that the metal, *lithium* protects against many toxins in brain cells, and using it during a three-month period boosts brain size by about two percent. Furthermore, the following has been reported in the scientific literature.

- Lithium is the biggest protector against toxins in brain cells, especially cellular garbage.
- Recovery from stroke with lithium in dogs is known to be effective.
- In Texas prison inmates, the higher the lithium dose, the less violence, rape, and suicide.
- As little as 20 mg lithium orotate or acetate purchased over the counter will protect neurons.

Prophylactically, I consume 120 mg lithium orotate tablets once weekly, and I combine it with other hormone therapies. This is what's new with my research.

Testosterone (T) also works by reducing *neural toxins* (beta-amyloid or brown cellular garbage) secreted in the brain during Alzheimer's. Also, Parkinson's increases the inflammatory factors (*cytokine*), and T alleviates them. In fact, T deficiency is known to cause *apathy* in Parkinson's disease (*J. Neurol. Neurosurg. Psychiatry*, 2004 Sept, 75(9), pp. 1323-1326). Through hormone replacement therapy, everyone *over fifty* should boost T, progesterone, and thyroid hormone back to levels of our youth if we want mental sharpness during our senior years. Many times I have seen older patients with some form of undiagnosed mental impairment. My knee-jerk reaction is to ask about their blood or urine levels of T, progesterone, cytokines (indicator of inflammation), and thyroid, if known.

In those over fifty, I often noticed minor mental malfunctions or adverse changes in temperament. I believe these changes are often attributable to low T, progesterone, and perhaps even thyroid hormone. Case study: Recently I met with a charming 50-year old lady known to be suffering from sub-clinical hypothyroidism (low thyroid hormone). This beautiful and intelligent woman resembled Angelina Jolie, and she was well educated with two university degrees. She arrived at our appointment after a long, exhausting walk. She felt chilled, and earlier in the day she had difficulties making decisions. I attempted to gain her attention without success.

Three times she failed to respond to my simple questions. Low thyroid hormone had shifted her brain into a temporary mental fog. She remained unaware of her attention deficit. See Table Two Chapter Five. She definitely needed an extra half grain of Armour® thyroid to carry her and her fogged brain through the day. This is a tragedy easily remedied with Armour. Standard blood tests for TSH (thyroid stimulating hormone) indicated her thyroid normal. Only a 24-hour urine test would reveal a significant shortfall of the most active of all thyroid hormones, called simply thyroid "T3." I have described this unfortunate lady's experience since many women over the age of 40 need *some extra* thyroid T3 for *optimal* brain efficiency. So called "normal" or "lower normal" brain function is not acceptable to me. You decide for yourself. Orthodox medicine would call her "normal" and not prescribe treatment. A pity.

This is the new finding of my research: pulling people from their mental fogs to more optimal brain efficiency. Also useful is supplementing some testosterone in all those deficient and over the age of fifty. In fact, to further verify my many observations, the May 2007 issue of *Archives of Neurology* describes a new successful treatment of *multiple sclerosis* or MS using 100 mg daily of testosterone cream. It works, and my theories are finally being vindicated in leading medical journals. Please try some Armour thyroid and testosterone yourself. What is wrong for performance-enhancing athletes has become right for seniors.

What a tragedy that Mother Nature has shortchanged us with hormone deficiencies during aging. We require them now just as in our youth since our body masses have remained relatively constant. Make no mistake. Becoming hormonally challenged is no fun.

Another Case Study
Eight percent of sixty-five year olds have some degree of senility, and this figure rises to 45% at age eighty.

Mr. Willis, 46, had been diagnosed with Parkinson's disease four years earlier. Thus far he had experienced mild symptoms of muscle rigidity, tremor, and slowed physical movement that had a devastating impact upon his everyday life. This terrible scourge commonly strikes older Americans with a host of disorders that eventually end in loss of physical movement, cognitive dysfunction, and death.

He became worried about mercury poisoning in his food since his naturopathic doctor believed that high mercury levels affected his Parkinson's. His own inquiries with Google revealed that mercury could cause mitochondrial damage.

He discovered that any level of mercury can harm a cell's mitochondria (*energy factories*), and that the severity of Parkinson's disease increased their dysfunction. No clinical studies clearly confirmed that enhancing mitochondrial function would mitigate the progression of his disease, but independent case studies suggested some benefit. Consequently, I recommended a regimen of CoQ10 supplementation to improve mitochondrial function. To chelate mercury from Mr. W's brain, I suggested *DMSA* as the agent of choice, as well as supplementing with l-glutathione and sublingual *Vitamin B-12*. Two grams daily of the anti-inflammatory spice, turmeric was also indicated. Several months later, Mr. Willis reported that this regimen did indeed mitigate his Parkinson's symptoms.

Vitamin B-12 remains critical to highly functioning and healthy brains. Healthy brains must also remain free of mercury and other heavy metals if one expects long life and mental health. Thus, to avoid mercury and other metal toxins, daily supplements of chelators such as DMSA become vital to any serious anti-aging regimen.

Now, I turn to my question posed in the title of this chapter, "Is Your Brain Receiving the Right Nutrients?" This question only matters if you want to live past sixty-five years of age with a healthy, sharp mind—not to mention avoiding depression, sleep disturbances, and weight gain. I have a number of friends in their sixties and seventies who complain of these symptoms, especially memory loss. And no wonder. *Eight percent of sixty-five year olds have some degree of senility, and this figure rises to 45% at age eighty.* But the worst effect is their gradual loss of personal identity that slowly slips away, especially with Alzheimer's where one becomes little more than a vegetable.

I first encountered this tragedy when I attended medical school at the University of Uppsala in Sweden. I remember visiting the geriatric ward as a young student where I was amazed to find most of the patients in a vegetative state. Through various forms of dementia, they were unable to care for their most elementary needs, such as going to the toilet and eating. The geriatric nurses needed only to hide the key to any particular door above the threshold. I asked why, and the nurses said that the patients lacked short-term memory needed to observe and remember the location of the keys. Their condition disheartened me, and I resolved to help alleviate it to the best of my ability. Some pop-culture authors have proposed that aging is "comfortable", but I categorically refute this myth due to my firsthand experiences with the uncomfortable tragedies of senility and aging.

At the other end of the spectrum, I married a young Swede who had a photographic memory. Her memory was so perfect that to this day she can still tell you word for word President Nixon's farewell address in the early 1970s. Word for word. She would often use this gift against me, remembering what I said in argument years earlier, which in turn forced me to improve my own memory in self-defense. As a result of her extraordinary gift, I became motivated in discovering why and how we gradually lose our memory and mental acuity during aging. Then I found how to improve my own memory and defend myself against verbal assaults.

Occasionally, I tried the prescription drug Diapid®, which diabetics used to control their flow of urine. Diapid has an interesting side effect. It raises short-term memory up to 50% during four-hour periods without harmful side effects since even weakened diabetic patients employ it. Using it allowed me to mount a moderate defense to my wife's perfect-memory assaults. Also, as a student, it helped me to study the nights before exams, which were often lengthy. All of these events piqued my interest in all forms of brain enhancements.

Preserving the Brain and Preventing Senility
A daily diet providing large quantities of fish oils allows the brain's neurons to regenerate themselves—not reproduce, regenerate.

Fresh unsaturated fish oils that have not become rancid are critical to health and longevity, especially in the human brain. Dr.

Nikola Scarmeas of Columbia University has reported in the *Annals of Neurology*, April, 2006, that diets low in animal fats and high in unsaturated oils from vegetable and *especially fish oils* reduced the chance of Alzheimer's disease by 40%. The exact reasons for this remain unknown, but I can make some educated guesses. From chemistry, I know the structure of these oils and their chemical fate in the body. From medicine, I know that a lack of fish oils may cause early onset of senility and even Alzheimer's. In between these two disciplines, lots of holes exist in our scientific knowledge. Interestingly, a diet rich in fish oils promotes regeneration of brain neurons —not reproduction, regeneration. Fresh, healthy fish oils contain the essential fatty acid *phosphatidylserine (PS)* that generates the successful transmission of electrical signals through the brain and out to the body's neurons. If one tries to regenerate neurons with land-animal fats or trans-fats, the results fail.

Both fish and vegetable oils have positive effects in human bodies and in all mammals. In particular, *fish oils* are extremely beneficial in maintaining healthy brains, spinal cords, and neural networks. Other good brain enhancers contain such nutrients as *coenzyme Q-10, turmeric, Vitamin B-12, vinpocetine, phosphatidylserine, thyroid, testosterone, progesterone, lithium,* and *acetyl-l-carnitine.* Several of these nutrients are reflected in my new research.

Therefore, I strongly recommend a diet *dominated* by fresh fatty fish, which contains high levels of *marine* omega-3-fatty acids. Notice that I have highlighted "marine" since this omega-3 is better than the vegetable types. All types supply essential building blocks in nerve cells which structurally allow nerve cell membranes a free flow of nutrients in and waste out. People with dementia do improve somewhat by taking these fish oil supplements and here again I am sure Mr. W would benefit. In other words, these supplements would provide Mr. Willis with needed nutritional support that would slow the deterioration of brain cells responsible for Parkinson's.

My own anecdotal study encompasses the aging population of Hawaii. When I encounter mentally alert seniors in their 70s or 80s, I will bet close friends that these seniors consume a high fish diet. I will ask and invariably confirm my assumption. Of course, in the case of those of Japanese ancestry, my friends will claim a cultural bias, but this does not refute the fact that they have made intelligent or fortunate choices about their diets. The same applies to elderly Anglos on the same diet.

A Scientific Demonstration of Dementia

The whys and wherefores of *dementia* are largely unknown. However, in recent decades some advances have been made by using special imaging techniques for viewing changes in healthy brains. One such technique employs PET or *positron emission tomography*. PET scans the brain and maps normal brain functions such as blood flow and cognitive activities. For example, in Alzheimer's disease, PET reveals decreases in brain metabolism as evidenced by declining use of oxygen and glucose. Other PET scans evaluate nerve receptors and their common nerve transmitters such as *dopamine* and *serotonin*. When using these tests, a mentally impaired brain reveals itself with darkened areas. On the other hand, enhanced brains show very brightly lighted areas, especially with over 100 mg daily of lithium. Interestingly, after only a three-week supplementation of 500 mg daily of the essential brain nutrients from fish, people with cognitive impairment light up like Christmas trees!

In other words, *impaired patients fed essential fish oil nutrients experienced brightened brains and enhanced mental activity.* Thus, I favor consuming a *heavy* fish diet or fish oil supplements.

So, eat your fish and maintain a healthy brain. *Fatty* fish such as salmon and herring offer special health advantages over *lean* fish such as tuna, cod, and fresh-water fish. But reversing years of consuming a diet of trans-fats remains impossible except through vacuuming one's thighs and stomach with liposuction. Older people who have consumed unhealthy fats for decades can perhaps benefit from an exercise program combined with lithium, hormonal, and chelation therapies as detailed later.

Some of my anti-aging patients say to me, "Dr. Lippman, I hate fish. Isn't there some other way?"

"Yes," I reply, "simply consume four grams per day of pure fish oil capsules free from PCBs, mercury, lead, and cadmium."

These capsules remain costly, but they will improve your health more than eating processed food. My dear friend, Dr. John Tonks suggested an alternative since he reframes from following his own patient advice or mine. He saves money by consuming daily two tablespoons of cod liver oil—exactly double the dose that his mother gave him as a child back in the 1930s in Merry Olde England. I have stood in his kitchen with a plate of brown beans on toast before me on the table. A proper English breakfast, what? Then John pulls out his little brown bottle of cod liver oil and takes a swig. It may be economical, but who really fancies the taste of it? Consequently, I encourage everyone to become a fresh-fish fanatic like myself and eat moderate portions daily. You will consume naturally all of the above nutrients and probably save yourself money. The result will be particularly pronounced if combined with some exercise along with this minor change in diet.

Note that I do not recommend radical diet changes such as fasting every other day. I do not recommend heavy exercise that generates eight times the amount of oxygen free radicals versus resting. These extreme remedies I leave to my celebrity competitors.

In addition to a hearty fresh-fish diet, one may supplement with weak antioxidants such as Vitamins A, C, D, and E and chelators such as the amino acids, l-glutathione and *DMSA* (*dimercapto succinic acid*). The latter helps with *autism*, especially if combined with 300mg daily of progesterone cream, since it "chelates" or eliminates heavy metals such as mercury from the brain and other tissues. Any sensible anti-aging program should employ some inexpensive *DMSA* and *l-glutathione*.

But beware, in 1998 while living in Hawaii, my blood contained three times the normal level of toxic mercury from eating cans of the predator fish tuna. I switched to a fresh diet of non-predator fish such as herring and salmon, and began taking 100 mg l-glutathione and 250 mg l-carnosine daily. Within a month, my blood mercury level dropped well below normal, and I felt great. This is what's new with my research. Obviously Mr. W also had this problem which may have contributed to his untimely Parkinson's.

Another nutrient critical to improving brain function and avoiding senility is Vitamin B-12. Vegetarians and the elderly lack it since they have difficulty either eating red meat or absorbing it through their intestines. Unfortunately, B-12's only natural source originates from red meat. People like me who consume low levels of red meat, or vegans and vegetarians who refuse it place themselves in harm's way, especially for senility. Believe me. Nearly half of all eighty year olds suffer from senility, and some senility becomes irreversible since the brain cannot tolerate a lifetime of nutritional abuse and then suddenly recover by some medical miracle. Damage is damage, and no force on this earth will change the situation. Science does not clearly understand why B-12 and other nutrients affect senility. By bridging chemistry, medicine, and physics, research will hopefully explain this connection in coming years.

My B-12 deficiency information sometimes upsets my vegetarian friends. They feel that they have discovered the ultimate diet for good health, and place great faith in the vegetarian lifestyle coupled with colonics and dietary fasting. I try to patiently hint that they really need some extra supplements when declining red meat. Often, they refuse to believe me, and their denial in the face of clear nutritional evidence endangers their brain health. They take pride in their beliefs, and who am I to dispute them? It reminds me of those who take pride in poverty. Since there is no nobility in poverty, there is no higher truth associated with the quasi-religious beliefs of strict vegans. I have offered a bet to my strict vegan friends. I will go with them to any health food store and pick out strict vegans and other non-meat eaters. The pallor of their skin reveals deficiencies of folic acid, iron, magnesium, and especially B-12. One can perhaps escape the most adverse effects of B-12 deficiency in one's youth, but when aging kicks in, deficiencies become all too apparent. Your health may suffer, especially your normal brain chemistry. And physicians cannot force people to be more responsible with their eating habits, except perhaps in Cuba. Who would want to fight the religion of vegetarianism anyway? Even public health authorities have no viable solutions for those unfortunates who refuse B-12.

A Scientific Demonstration of B-12 Deficiencies

For example, if you take a blood test for B-12 in the U.S., an American lab will declare your B-12 level to be "normal" if it falls within the range of 200 to 1100 pg/ml. However, most foreign labs have higher standards. Japanese labs declare normal to be from 500 to 1300 pg/ml, and Swedish labs declare the healthy range to fall between 1000 to 3000 pg/ml. This means that your U.S. lab and physician may tell you that you are normal when in fact you are headed for irreversible senility due to lack of B-12. This is my original research. *In the U.S., the problem with many other so-called normal lab values is that they are based upon blood tests from the sick and elderly!* These so-called normal values may shorten your life, and/or cost you irreparable brain damage. More accurate assessments of normal values of minimum 600 pg/ml should be determined from the blood tests of young, healthy adults in their twenties or thirties. In Sweden, labs collect many truly healthy blood values from recruits to the Swedish army—typically young men nineteen to twenty-one years of age.

As in the case of melatonin, you should not rely on consuming B-12 *oral supplements.* They do not absorb well since they must bind with an intrinsic factor in the intestine's *duodenum.* Instead, try B-12 injections or nasal spray. My favorite third choice not requiring an intrinsic factor is sublingual methyl B-12 (available at www.vrp.com). You can also try eye-dropping the liquid or crushing the tablets between your teeth and allowing it to absorb under the tongue for a few minutes. Sublingual administration also works well with many hormone supplements.

I personally eat only small portions of red meat once or twice a month, and in between I supplement with methyl B-12. In addition, one should consume daily 50 mg Vitamin B-6, 0.8 mg folate, 1 gram *magnesium gluconate* and not its oxide form, and/or 50 mg *TMG* (*tri-methyl glycine*). All of these will help to lower your *fibrinogen*, a key indicator of Alzheimer's disease.

Orthodox medicine often ignores many key supplements critical to any serious anti-aging program. Well-meaning medical practitioners trained only in diseases should not be faulted since conventional medical schools do have their limits. Other nutrients designated as normal by the U.S., but not by foreign labs will be discussed later.

The Miracle of Centrophenoxine
Scientists call this lifetime storage of oxidized garbage MICROINSULTS—the chemical ones, not the verbal ones.

Oxidation and free-radical attacks also cause another type of damage called *lipofuscin*, or *age pigment* as a result of an inflammatory process. Large quantities of age pigment occur in the brains of people suffering from Alzheimer's, and when seen on the skin of the elderly, age pigment is popularly called "*age spots.*" *During aging, every cell naturally accumulates age pigment in amounts equal to one third or more of a cell's total volume.* This is yet another one of Mother Nature's many dirty tricks played during the aging process. We really only notice some age pigment-clogged brown cells on the surface of our aging skin, but in reality, millions of other hidden cells throughout our body also become clogged with the same garbage during aging. Scientists call this lifetime storage of oxidized garbage *microinsults*—the chemical ones, not the verbal ones.

Enter the miracle nutrient *centrophenoxine*, which gradually removes age pigment without covering them up cosmetically with make-up or bleaching. Your typical American physician will not recognize this unique nutrient developed by me and others in Europe. Indeed, in France and some other European countries, one can purchase it over-the-counter in some pharmacies. Centrophenoxine should be a core element in anyone's anti-aging and optimal health program. It increases the brain's use of glucose and improves brain energy levels. It also removes excessive potassium build-up in the brain as well as in the heart, lungs, and skin cells. It properly balances potassium and sodium, and their transfer across cell membranes. Dating back to 1982, I have personally researched centrophenoxine and its close cousin DMAE, and I tested and confirmed their cellular "garbage removal" qualities. I have used it in my own anti-aging regimen and have often recommended it.

While living and traveling in Europe during those years, I occasionally met people interested in anti-aging remedies. If they were at least middle age and older, I could usually observe their first signs of aging which included graying hair and age spots on their hands, arms, and sometimes even on their faces. While explaining anti-aging treatments, I diplomatically asked my newfound acquaintances if they would like to remove their age spots without surgery or bleaching. This is my new research. If interested, I sent them to a local pharmacy asking for centrophenoxine. Upon a later encounter, they usually thanked me profusely for my help. I am always glad to be of help for those seeking anti-aging advice. Centrophenoxine should be sourced from Europe through www.antiaging-motivate.com. Its benefits are largely unknown to American physicians unless knowledgeable in anti-aging medicine.

Centrophenoxine is also known to prevent intellectual deterioration and to increase storage of new information into long-term memory. Increased vigilance and alertness occurs after only a few weeks of treatment since it reverses age-related drops in brain proteins. For the best effect in the brain, please take on an empty stomach before one eats a large fish meal.

In summary, remember that no one wants a rancid brain. See figure below. On the other hand, consuming 250 mg daily of centrophenoxine removes age pigment in skin cells and throughout the body. I take 250 mg daily. Who needs their cells clogged with oxidized age pigment debris?

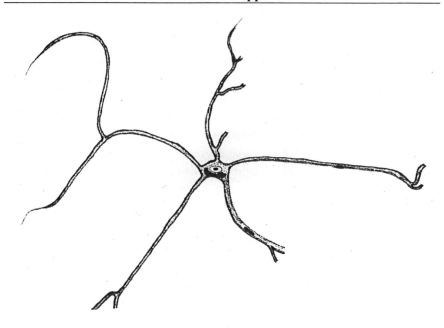

Figure 1. An aging neuron from the human spinal cord. The black spots are lipofuscin or age pigment that accumulates gradually and deposits itself in the neuron's *perikaryon* and *dendritic* branches. *One third or more of a cell's volume eventually fills with age pigment during aging.* This effect is believed to slow transmission of nerve signals and to hinder transport of nutrients and wastes to and from various neurons.

Keeping Your Aging Brain Flexible, Spontaneous & Curious
"We don't stop playing because we grow old; we grow old because we stop playing." George Bernard Shaw

Even if aging brains exhibit no symptoms of senility, they may become more inflexible during aging, and science does not exactly understand why this occurs. My best guess leans toward a deficiency of essential brain nutrients commonly available in a high fish diet. By inflexibility I mean an inability to adapt to new ideas in an ever changing modern world. If you remain unconvinced, consider how many older people you know who cannot use a computer or learned everyday information needed in today's modern world. Despite federal laws against age discrimination, people whose inflexible minds prevent them from adapting to new circumstances have a difficult time adjusting to a modern world. When I see this phenomenon in friends and patients, I realize that they need help, and without it, future senility may result. A pity.

Picasso Lends a Hand

The primary symptom of an aging brain, long before signs of senility become apparent, is an inability to flexibly change and adapt to one's environment.

Flexibility and continued adjustment to society's demands are essential for a happy, prosperous life, and a senility-free brain. One intriguing example I borrowed from Françoise Gillot's book, *Matisse and Picasso*. Picasso's youngest son Claude, a five year old, sat and drew at the feet of Henri Matisse. Upon completion, Claude signed his drawing Claude Matisse and handed it to Henri. The artist was taken aback. He asked the boy why he refused to sign it Claude Picasso, since Picasso is a perfectly good artist name. Claude replied that his father acted childish and insincere. In later years, Claude never became a great artist like his father Pablo Picasso, who retained his childish and insincere artistic temperament well into his eighties and nineties. Seriousness and rigidity towards art or life did not seem to help Claude. Apparently, light-heartedness, flexibility, spontaneity, and curiosity reflect essential keys not only to longevity but a creative and healthy brain as well. This is my new research that I call "The Picasso Paradigm" which means that the primary symptom of an aging brain, long before signs of senility become apparent, is an inability to flexibly change and adapt to one's environment.

The Picasso Paradigm reflects the importance of maintaining a sense of humor throughout life. New York socialite Mrs. Brooke Astor lived to 105 years old and always maintained a strong sense of humor. She once said that "unlike Queen Victoria, we *are* amused – we are always amused". Mrs. Astor's commitment to humor is surely a vital key to a long life. I agree.

Sites/ Causes of Mitochondrial Dysfunction \ Nutrients That Normalize Mitochondrial Bioenergetics	Co Q10	Idebenone	ALC	NAC	Lipoic Acid	Omega 3 FAs	Vitamin B1	Vitamin B2	Vitamin B3	Ginkgo Biloba	Succinic Acid	Exercise
Complex I	X						X	X			X	
Complex II	X							X			X	
Complex III	X											
Complex IV				X							X	
Complex V				X							X	
Membrane Potential			X		X							
Membrane Cardiolipin			X			X						
Coenzyme Q10 Level	X		X									
Carnitine Level			X									
ATP Biosynthesis	X				X							
Fatty Acid Transport			X									
Cellular Respiration			X	X	X				X			X
Antioxidant	X			X[1]	X[2,3]	X				X		X[2,4]
Reduces Lactic Acid	X						X				X	
Improves Muscle Strength	X				X							X
Decreases Muscle Fatiguability	X				X							X
Improves Cognition		X	X									
Increases Neurotransmitters			X									
Improves Receptor Sensitivity			X									
Increases Phosphatidylcholine						X						
Increases Pyruvic Acid							X					

Table 1. Nutrients that normalize mitochondria function. (Supplied by Ward Dean, MD).

CoQ10 and Parkinson's
This nutrient is more important to your future health than even a daily multiple vitamin supplement.

Enter the eminent cardiologist, Dr. Stephen Sinatra, who is no relation to Frank, but is just as much of a star to all longevity docs. Dr. Sinatra's heart patients consume at least 400 mg daily of coenzyme Q-10 or *CoQ10* to improve energy and health of mitochondria in the heart and other organs. I recommend 2,400 mg daily in Parkinson's to reduce brain deterioration since my research dating from 1983 indicated significant benefits from CoQ10.

CoQ10 is a viscous orange liquid extracted from beef heart. I have always considered this nutrient to be vital to the brain and heart and have recommended it to everyone serious about anti-aging therapy. The latest CoQ10 news reports that a better version called

Idebenone has arrived in the marketplace. You know that this one helps your body since its primary use has been the preservation of harvested transplant organs. It works.

Interestingly, human aging is often defined as the loss of cells in every organ throughout the body. For this reason, our muscles lose half their strength between the ages of thirty-five and seventy, and this effect can *partially* be remedied by regular exercise. Obviously, an excellent anti-aging regimen would include at least 150 mg daily of CoQ10 and double that if you have heart disease or take statin drugs, and in the case of Parkinson's, 1,200 to 2,400 mg. After about a month, those who forget this critical nutrient become tired and lethargic. Please remember to take this nutrient. It is more important to your future health than even a daily multiple vitamin supplement. If you must miss one or the other, then please drop the multiple vitamin supplements.

The Lippman 3-Step Brain Program for Maintaining Brain Health
Used in Combination with Plans A, B, or C.
Patient empowerment is critical.

An enormous variety of brain enhancers are available, and the question arises of what should an ordinary person passing middle age take assuming limited aging symptoms and a limited budget? Nutrient costs and patient empowerment remain critical. I recommend a daily practice following my 3-step Brain Program combined with previously mentioned anti-aging Plans A, B, and C. Take the following supplements divided up into a maximum of six capsules or tablets during daily meals. All of these supplements should be taken on an empty stomach, and then one should sit down to eat a balanced, healthy meal.

● **Step One for Those on a Tight Budget** of about a dollar a day. *A strong diet dominated by fresh fish* or fish-oil capsules. If at least 20% of your total calories originate from fish, your metabolism will rise by about 15%. (My research) Also, try taking daily supplements of 2 mg Vitamin B-12 sublingually, 50 mg B-6, min. 150 mg CoQ10 or Idebenone, and mixing your morning fruit juice (*grapefruit* or *pomegranate*) together with a tablespoon of Mitoboost I and II available at www.vrp.com.

A*:* Add another fifty cents daily. *For those experiencing memory fade*, try 2.5 to 5 mg once or twice daily of Hydergine™. I have used this since 1982, and I know that boring tasks such as long distance night driving are more easily performed at a higher level of attention. Another over-the-counter alternative employs the hormone pregnenolone. Take 100 mg daily in the morning for four months and then 50 mg per day when memory fading symptoms improve.

B: Add another two dollars daily. *For those experiencing brain-fog*, I have four suggestions. First try a half grain daily of Armour® thyroid. For further sharpening, try Diapid®. Since 1982, I have sprayed in my nose single doses of lysine-vasopressin or trade named Diapid®. (My research) As a natural hormone, it eliminates brain fog and increases short-term memory by 25% to 50% for a four-hour period. It is a great little pick-me-up for students. For older folks, I would suggest *Piracetam* or its analogues, *Aniracetam* or the latest, *Pramiracetam*. (www.antiaging-motivate.com). These smart drugs or nootropics are safe and increase communication across the brain's *corpus callosum* and also remove brain fog and increase IQ, in which the person already has a high I.Q. Lastly, my best alternative remedy employs vitamins: Try consuming 200 mg B2 and 500 mg B3 daily, and within hours of the first dose, all symptoms of brain fog will clear, concentration will improve, and energy will normalize.

C: Add another 30 cents daily. *For those concerned with pre-Alzheimer's,* try two to three grams daily of turmeric. Turmeric or curcumin is the yellow color in curry spice. It helps immune cells clean out of amyloid-beta plaques in your brain.

• **Step Two for Those with Disposable Income**. Add another two dollars daily. If you absolutely refuse to eat a diet that consists of a lot of fresh fish and must instead use substitutes such as *fish oil capsules*, try adding daily to step one such brain nutrients as 10 mg *vinpocetine*, 250 mg *centrophenoxine* and 200 mg *phosphatidylserine*.

A: Add another 20 cents daily. *For those experiencing anxiety*, add 150 to 300 mg daily *l-theanine*, kava, or St. John's Wort. L-theanine is a natural amino acid and my favorite.

B: Add another 50 cents daily. *For those experiencing depression and poor sleep* patterns, try adding to the above 0.5 mg melatonin crushed and positioned under the tongue one hour before bedtime. This works best sublingually along with some other hormones. Also recommended at bedtime is 500 mg of *l-tryptophan* or *100mg bio-identical progesterone (P) cream plus 0.5 mg melatonin rubbed into the scalp (my research)*. Women may take up to 300 mg P daily, while men with erection problems should reduce this dose to only 15 to 30 mg daily. Alternatively, see a physician knowledgeable in anti-aging medicine and take a 24-hour urine test: Your poor sleep may also be resulting from other hormone problems such as too low or high cortisol.

- **Step Three for the Well Healed.** Costs here vary widely between $500 to 1,000 monthly depending upon your physician's recommendations. For the truly adventurous and for those worried about *memory loss and attention failure*, I strongly recommend partnering with a health care professional, especially one knowledgeable in anti-aging medicine. These professionals can advise you on further testing and the suitability of such enhancers as pyritinol, Deprenyl, deaner, Huperzine-A, inositol, GABA, tryptophan, choline, manganese, taurine, other B vitamins, branched-chain amino acids, l-dopa, phenylalanine, tyrosine, yohimbine, chromium, lithium, the sex hormones, thyroid hormone, and many other anti-aging drugs and nutrients. However, my absolute daily favorite remains consuming fish supported by a half grain Armour thyroid and 100 mg of bio-identical testosterone cream.

Further Thoughts about the Brain
The Lippman 3-step Brain Program uniquely encourages everyone in getting started even if they have limited knowledge of anti-aging medicine.

Brain enhancers are a difficult subject both to understand and employ. I only know that they really work from personal experiences without resorting to prescription anti-depressants and sleep aids. For example, a good friend of mine gave brain enhancers to his children, and when one boy was four years old, his photo and story ended up in the national tabloid press since the boy could fully operate a computer.

My own justification came when I visited my friend Dr. Glenn Braswell, chief editor at the *Journal of Longevity* in the early 1990s. He had called me to his office for a discussion of anti-aging and longevity. He engaged me in an intriguing conversation for almost an hour. He was amazed to learn that I had an anti-aging product registered by the Italian FDA and sold at the Vatican's only pharmacy. He later confirmed this and the Pope's blessing on a visit to Rome. Eventually his employee interrupted us with a company budget sheet. The sheet listed a large set of subscriber numbers and payments of subscription fees. He wanted some totals which his employee could not supply. Then he ordered a calculator. I offered to give him the totals without a calculator. Ever since my experiences with brain-enhancement nutrients, I could easily multiply and divide sundry lists of figures in my head. I gave Braswell the totals he sought within in a few minutes. He beamed with surprise and wanted me to write an article about my brain-enhancing regimen. I thanked him for his compliment which I had always perceived as a schoolboy's trick. I believed that many others could do this trick, especially if trained as accountants or engineers and if properly enhanced.

I encourage everyone to empower themselves with the Lippman 3-step Brain Program as well as other nutrients in this book. Many authors neglect to explain how to implement their recommendations. They leave the reader flat-footed. The Lippman 3-step Brain program uniquely encourages everyone to get started even if they have limited knowledge of anti-aging medicine. Starting my program is especially important in avoiding diseases of the brain as explained in this chapter's beginning with Mr. Willis. Furthermore, you should get at least seven hours of sleep nightly which keeps your cortisol and inflammation at bay. All this will result in a healthier brain and a happier person. You will feel better with more vitality and energy than you thought possible. Life becomes an exciting adventure again.

Recommendations

Additional tips to the Lippman 3-Step Brain Program.

- Fifteen percent of your diet dominated by fresh or lightly pan-seared fish or fish oil capsules or cod liver oil (*marine omega-3 fatty acids*).
- Cut back or eliminate caffeine and alcohol. These raise the stress hormone, cortisol and nearly double the amount of unwanted estrogens in men.
- For men only: *smaller* portions of veggies than women eat, and nuts & seeds plus a fish- dominant diet. For women only: Any amount of veggies & vegetable oil products and fish-dominant diet. Do not use corn oil or high fructose corn syrup lavishly applied in food at many chain coffee houses and restaurants.
- Minimum 7 hours sleep nightly with 0.5 mg melatonin and 100 mg (women) or 30 mg (men) progesterone. Your longevity will decrease significantly if you do not sleep at least 7 hours nightly. Also, a minimum of 30 minutes exercise daily. One and a half hours of exercise daily is optimal.
- Maintain a flexible, spontaneous, curious, fun-loving, amused attitude even in your senior years.
- Men over 50 use testosterone replacement therapy daily and post-menopausal women use estradiol, estriol, and at least 100 mg progesterone daily. (100 mg three times daily for female problems.)
- Blood tests are quick and easy and paid for by insurance, but they often are insufficient in determining multiple hormone shortages and their remedies. Instead, I always recommend testing all 29 of your hormones and their metabolites with a

24-hour urine test available at www.meridianvalleylab.com. Armed with this test, knowledgeable anti-aging physicians can help you with improved brain function and better sleep. These tests are the cutting edge of anti-aging technology since they have only been available to the general public during recent years.

Golden Key to Longevity #7

- *The brain is composed of seventy percent fat. If you chose to fill it with a lifetime of hamburger oils* and trans-fats, it may refuse to function well in your senior years with an ability to make flexible changes. Thus long before senility becomes apparent, a primary symptom may be an inability to flexibly make changes and adapt to an ever changing world. Be flexible and amused; always be amused by life.*

*A very well known Hollywood actor often eats hamburgers at 3 am and his male-menopause waistline reveals this damaging habit. It is also bad for retaining a healthy brain into one's senior years.

APPENDIX A
For those with additional *brain*-function problems:

- *Brain exercises* with puzzles or learning a new skill are essential in maintaining a sharp mind well into one's eighties and nineties. One should exercise the brain at least two hours a day if one hopes to retain mental acuity in decades to follow.

- *For brain protection*, one needs to consume at least twice daily *strong* antioxidants such as l-glutathione or methionine that further strengthen our lines of defense against free radicals. And by strong antioxidants, I definitely do not mean *weak* Vitamins C, D, and E.

- *For enhanced brain and body function*, one ought to consume mitochondrial boosters such as Dr. Ward Dean's *Mitoboost One and Two* available from www.vrp.com. Please check out the enormous body of research at this site. Briefly, Mitoboost supplements facilitate and increase mitochondrial health, energy, membrane potential, cognitive performance, production of neural transmitters, sensitivity of hormone receptors, quenching of free radicals, and better use of mitochondrial oxygen.

- *For better arterial support to the brain*, I advise 10 mg daily of vinpocetine available from www.Swansonvitamins.com. Briefly, vinpocetine is the only nutrient that improves cerebral metabolism and blood flow, especially in the microcirculation of small arteries. It enhances brain-cell ATP production, neural transmitter turnover, and brain utilization of oxygen and glucose. I also strongly endorse a cup daily of pomegranate juice.

- *For increasing brain-cell energy and preventing stroke* from one of the oldest of the smart drugs, I advise at least 100 mg daily of *pyritinol* and 250 to 500 mg daily of DMAE or *centrophenoxine* available from www.antiaging-motivate.com. Still another old time standby is the brain-supporting drug *Hydergine*®.

- *For positive benefits to memory, brain longevity, and mood*, I advise 200 mg daily of *phosphatidylserine or PS*, along with pyritinol. PS increases brain acetylcholine and oxygen.

- *For better focus and concentration*, I recommend the simple amino acid *l-theanine*. L-theanine has some anti-obesity properties, and it is an excellent way to reduce irritability. I take 150 mg when anxious, while my Jack Russell terrier gets 20 mg for occasional bouts of separation anxiety. The pet version is available at 1800Petmeds.com.

- *For both protection and enhancement*, I strongly advise consuming a minimum of 200 mg daily of *Coenzyme Q-10* or *Idebenone*, available at some pharmacies and health food stores. Also, I encourage 100 mg daily of *R- lipoic acid.*

- *For clearing the brain of cellular garbage* that clogs brain cells, I strongly advise using bio-identical testosterone, estradiol, estriol, and progesterone creams available from compounding pharmacies and not their drug equivalents. For shrinking brains and recovery from stroke, one could consume 240 mg of lithium two or three times daily available over the counter in many pharmacies. Also highly recommended is prophylactic use of a half grain daily of Armour® thyroid hormone.

Section 2

The Lippman Plan

This section begins by outlining a simple step-by-step approach to implementing my anti-aging recommendations. I have divided the plan into three levels of usage depending upon reader requirements and finances. I designed this plan for middle-aged people and older without memory problems. Memory issues were addressed separately in Chapter 7. Lastly, everything new and unique to my research is highlighted in italics below.

My oldest son read the following three plans and asked me if only the rich can afford anti-aging medicine. No, I replied. Plan A requires a budget of less than fifty dollars monthly and some will power to resist modern American eating habits. Plan B can be implemented on less than eighty dollars a month without major lifestyle changes such as visits to 24-hour sweat palaces or radical new diets. However, plan C may well cost 500 to 800 dollars monthly, and it is only recommended to the well heeled and for those committed to slowing their aging and the associated adult-onset diseases of aging -- the pre-diseases often ignored by orthodox medicine.

Chapter References

Plan A: Desire some changes, but not ready to overhaul their lives.

Chapters 1, 3, 5, 6

1. *One pill/one meal daily (d) of truly strong antioxidants: l-glutathione, l-methionine, BHT, NDGA, and/or DMSA.*
2. *Minimum 150 mg/d CoQ10 and 12.5 mg/d iodine tablets.*
3. 5,000 IU/d Vitamin D3 or about 35,000 IU weekly. Wash it down with pomegranate juice.
4. Try to cut back on all forms of sugar which means avoiding many American foods.
5. *Please consume fish or fish oil capsules daily. Fatty fish such as salmon and mackerel are the best source for marine omega threes.*

Plan B: Desire changes, but wish to retain basic lifestyle.

Chapters 1, 2, 5, 6, 7, 8

1. Implement plan A.

2. Substitute all forms of sugar for xylitol sugar using twice as much as ordinary sugar.
3. Avoid caffeine and milk products: substitute with decaf and some soy milk.
4. *Consume fresh fish or fish oil capsules up to an optimal 15% of total dietary intake.*
5. *Consume one capsule DMSA after every fish meal.*
6. *Consume 2 grams/d turmeric,* 1 gram/d magnesium gluconate (not oxide), 50 mg/d R-lipoic acid, 30 mg/d resveratrol.
7. Weekly or biweekly oral chelation with 6 caps Oral ChelatoRx™ (vrp.com).
8. *Daily consumption of anti-cross linkers such as 150mg/d aminoguanidine or Metformin™ and 500 mg/d l-carnosine.*

Plan C: Desire complete lifestyle makeover for max effect.

Chapters 5 thru 19

1. Implement plans A and B.
2. Do blood, saliva, and *24-hr urine tests* with the help of a knowledgeable anti-aging physician.
3. Correct hormone deficiencies with bio-identical hormone replacement therapy (BHRT): testosterone for men and women, estradiol plus progesterone for women. HGH injections and Armour® thyroid tablets for both men and women especially if over the age of fifty. Use aldosterone and progesterone for those who are deficient. Men: Avoid enlarged prostate with 30 mg/d bio-identical progesterone applied every morning to the genitals. Women: Avoid cardiovascular and other aging diseases by daily replacement with bio-identical estradiol, progesterone, testosterone, estriol, etc. as indicated by blood or 24-hour urine tests. Men: Avoid cardiovascular and other aging diseases by daily reinstatement with bio-identical testosterone cream or gel, 50 to 100 mg/d; plus Armour thyroid. Especially test FREE T3 (the biologically active thyroid hormone) with 24-hour urine test three times annually.
4. Correct dietary deficiencies, especially Vitamin B12, folate, magnesium, and minerals. Test annually or semi-annually for deficiencies, especially in regard to amino acids.

5. In case of elevated blood pressure or claudication (peripheral vascular disease), use IV chelation weekly for at least 20 weeks. Detoxify brain and other tissues with oral DMSA therapy, *especially with every fish meal.*

6. If needed, use special enzyme blockers as determined by 24-hr urine tests.

7. Trust your knowledgeable anti-aging physician. Test annually for C-reactive protein, Hb-A1c, fibrinogen, etc.

Chapter 8
The Man Who Would Cheat Death

Regenerative Tissues and Renewable Skin and Organs
"Good medical care can influence which direction a person's old age will take. Give us a disease, and we can do something about it. Most of us in medicine, however, don't know how to think about decline. But give us an elderly woman with [multiple aliments of aging], and we are not sure about what to do".
Harvard Professor A. Gawande

In 2007 I met my friend, Harvard trained Jonathan Wright, MD and his lovely wife Holly at an International Hormone Society conference in Los Angeles. Jonathan explained to me his success with treating a handful of patients in his Kent, Washington clinic with the hormone, *aldosterone (A)*. Anecdotal evidence suggests that a deficiency of A is responsible for some types of hearing loss. I was mesmerized by this new piece of research since I had inherited *tinnitus* from my father and grandfather. This meant that I had some hearing loss after passing middle age, especially in the range of 4,000 to 8,000 Hertz, where half my hearing had vanished at age 59 as in the case of my ancestors. In fact, at age 75 my father had lost eighty percent of his hearing in this range.

Consequently, I followed Jonathan's expert advice and began taking 125 micrograms of A twice daily. After the first month, no effects were apparent. Then two weeks later I was walking in the Broadway area of New York City, and something dramatic happened. In narrow streets with high building, the noises of passing cars and trucks became incredibly irritating to me. I was forced to wear protective ear-gear, and I realized that my hearing had changed, but I remained unconvinced if these changes were for the better. Walking the streets of mid-town Manhattan was like wearing an iPod with the sound turned-up full volume and an earpiece glued in my ear!

Upon returning home, I noticed that the volume control on my radio required only a normal 18 to 22 setting on a maximum 60 scale, and this had significantly changed from a setting of 28 to 35 two months previously. Something marvelous had happened to my hearing, and I sought further measurements from the local audiologist who had tested me three years ago. He retested my hearing and discovered it had changed from a fifty percent loss to a thirty-one percent loss in the range of 4,000 to 8,000 Hertz. Secondly, my night blindness while driving or walking seemed to improve. Thirdly, my symptoms of jet lag disappeared by about 80%, especially when traveling through many time zones from west to east. As a result of these revelations, I enthusiastically applied my research skills and sought to acquire as much knowledge as possible about this wonderful hormone. My inquiries led me to the following information.

Aldosterone is known to regulate kidney function and plays a critical role in potassium and sodium balance which induces a positive voltage of at least 80 millivolts in the nerves of the inner ear and in other nerve sensors in the head. Doctors D. Trune and J. Kempton (Hearing Research, 2001; 155(1-2): 9-20) found that aldosterone (A) combined with *pregnisolone*, restored auditory function in lab mice due to increasing sodium transport and positive voltage in the inner ears' *stria vascularis.* A team of researchers in New York have reported that *patients with severe hearing loss had half as much aldosterone compared to people with normal hearing.*

Still other researchers report that good vision depends upon adequate supplies of A combined with a minimum amount of the hormone *cortisol*. Those with blurred vision as a result of aging may have deficient A which restricts Vitamin A's function for normal vision. In my case, daily supplementation of A has resulted in enhanced night vision. Lack of night vision or *nyctalopia* means that the aging rods of the eyes restrict detection of weak light of semi-darkness. Aldosterone seems to enhance night vision much like nocturnal cats that have exceptional night vision. I have found myself walking in semi-darkness at night without needing artificial lighting. I believe it. During aging, one can maintain good hearing and vision only if one has an adequate supply of hormones such as aldosterone, cortisol and perhaps a little pregnisolone. I came to realize that after the age of 50, many people are hormonally challenged and they may well benefit from supplementing several different hormones in balanced symphony.

In conclusion, I have enormous faith in Dr. Wright, and I personally take aldosterone 120 micrograms twice daily to alleviate tinnitus, night blindness, and even my jet lag. In regard to the latter, I can now fly through twelve time zones with only minor drowsiness upon arriving at my destination. Without aldosterone replacement therapy, I was incapacitated with sleepiness at the rate of one sleepy day for every hour of time-zone change. Aldosterone capsules and bio-identical creams are only available at Key Pharmacy in Kent, WA. www.keynutritionrx.com. This is truly the cutting-edge bio-identical hormone replacement therapy of the future, and I believe that Dr. Wright and others have stumbled upon a remarkable advancement in anti-aging therapy. Go for it.

New body parts needed during aging
Aging takes its mechanical toll on our bodies.

I wrote this chapter with the idea that people require new body parts during aging, especially if they neglect to maintain their organs and cells with the nutrients delineated in this book. In the distant future this might be achieved with stem cells developing into individual organ tissues that replace worn-out organs. Stem cell research has not advanced to this stage of development yet and may never, especially if our political leaders refuse to support basic science and research due to their personal beliefs. Without advances in stem cells and organ/tissue replacement, the old fashion, more mundane methods remain such as replacement with stainless steel balls in Teflon sockets used in hip surgery. Acquiring new parts does not mean one stops taking vitamins, nutrients, and vital hormones such as testosterone, progesterone, and thyroid hormone. Unfortunately, some body parts wear out no matter how much or how often one takes hormones and strong antioxidants. Aging takes its *mechanical* toll on our bodies, and some aspects of aging can be prevented or reversed with various supplements, but others must be replaced. Ask any dentist. Teeth will only last fifty plus years, and mechanical wear and tear and even peritonitis compels us to visit a friendly dentist. Other examples include the mechanical wearing-out of hip joints.

I myself have never needed any body part replacements or even surgery since I have always taken care of myself with the right nutrients, be they vitamins, minerals, hormones, or powerful free-radical scavengers. This simple fact really floors many physicians. But perhaps I have been lucky, and I admit that I am a cockeyed optimist, largely due to euphoria encouraged by daily natural testosterone replacement therapy described in detail in the following two chapters. Optimistically, I see no limits to restricting the wear and tear of my own body as long as I persist with a serious anti-aging program. As reported in an earlier chapter, I am lacking in wear and tear and benefiting physically by dancing the twist down to the one foot level of a limbo stick – much like I have always done since my teenage years. But, I must admit that others remain largely indifferent to their health until a disease strikes. Therefore, they may eventually require some surgical help when approaching their senior years, if not earlier. Take notice, aging becomes a terrible task master, and my competitors who often write about the joys of menopause, old age, and shuffleboard, seem a bit silly. Allow me to explain some examples of my friends who deny anti-aging medicine and then require new body parts. Take Bill Benson, age sixty three.

Bill needed a hip replacement, and he sought the cheapest hip parts possible with the help of his Navy pension. The mother of another friend, Birgit needed a new hip and placed herself on an eighteen-month waiting list – such are the problems with Medicaid, or in other countries with socialized medicine. Another dear friend in his seventies required laser cataract surgery. He was unwilling to investigate the patented Russian eye drops that would have repaired his lenses without surgery. In other words, most people will require some form of body part replacement if they live long enough and avoid anti-aging therapy as advocated in this book. Consequently, I obliged my friends by trying to source the right parts and hold their hands during surgery and recovery. Compassion and empathy remain paramount when dealing with the disabilities of aging.

Renewable Eyes
"She slept with an ophthalmologist who kept asking, 'Is it better like this, or like this?"
Russell T. Stoddard, MD

The eyes do deteriorate as we age, and without surgical substitutions available such as artificial or cadaver eye-replacement, we must wait another twenty years for scientists to grow new eyes in a Petri dish. Let us review briefly what aging does to the eyes.

A Scientific Explanation for Aging Eyes

During the aging of a healthy sixty year old, the amount of light reaching the eyes' interior retina is about one third what you would find in the eyes of a healthy twenty year old. The eye's retina contains two types of photoreceptors, namely rods and cones, which provide us with vision and allow us to see fine details in this book. The rods remain essential for night vision and motion detection since they are more sensitive than cones during the night and conditions of dim lighting. A second component called the iris controls light passing into the interior of the eyes. Tiny muscles on the side of the iris control its opening and closing which weakens during aging and prevents the admission of necessary light. Thus a loss of vision occurs since the iris cannot open sufficiently to allow in needed light, especially under weak lighting conditions. This condition reminds me of reading in a darkened room with sunglasses. Second to the weakening of iris muscles is the loss of rods as we age.

The rods of the eyes detect weak light, and such animals as cats have many more of them than humans which allow them better vision in the dark. Young humans have at least nine times as many rods as cones, but during aging our number of cones remains unchanged while our number of rods decreases by about one third. The loss of rods and the weakening of iris muscles account for aging, and therefore, humans have difficulty adjusting to varying intensities of light from passing cars during night driving.

Free radicals and cross linking causes the clouding of the lens of the eyes as we age, especially with sun exposure like one experiences in sunny states. In other words, a lifetime of free-radical attack and cross linking causes cataract formation. Until recently cataracts could only be corrected by surgery since antioxidants cannot reach the lenses which lack supporting blood vessels. In my case I have always supplied my body with strong antioxidants carried by my arteries to nearly all tissues in my body, except to the inaccessible lenses of the eyes. Thus, my lenses were aging much more rapidly than my body. I had forgotten this simple fact. Then Russian scientists invented special anti-glycation drops specifically for the inaccessible lenses. Thanks to these advances, I welcome you to 21st century medicine that allows cataracts, and especially pre-cataracts, to be gradually reversed.

New Cure for Cataracts without Laser Surgery
I found myself reading price tags and debit-card terminals without needing glasses.

Cataract surgery belongs to the past. Anyone who adamantly and categorically denies this fact is either uninformed or opting for the surgical fees. In the specialty of anti-aging medicine, something remarkable has happened in recent years – similar to finding the monolith on the moon in the film, "2001 Space Odyssey." A cure has been found for cataracts and some related aging-eye phenomena that promises to relegate many eye surgeries to the dustbin of medical history. But unfortunately our benevolent FDA has yet to approve it. For the thousands of victims of premature loss of vision, it holds an open door and a promise of new sight where only the cloudiness of vision reigned before. An outstanding research team of Russian scientists led by Dr. M. A. Babizhayev has invented this new cure. Historically, a Russian team should be unsurprising since another Russian research team invented *radial keratotomy* back in the nineteen seventies. Radial keratotomy means the radial cutting of the outside rim of the lens with a fine surgical knife. American know-how eventually modified this procedure by substituting a fine-cutting laser for a surgical knife, and it became known as "laser eye surgery" which we all take for granted today.

Back in 1981 I worked as a researcher at the Department of Medical Cell Biology in Sweden, and I mentored under a professor of histology who also practiced as an eye doctor one day a week in order to relieve long lines of eye patients needing treatment in Sweden's socialized-medical care. I asked him what he thought of a new method, "radial keratotomy", commonly used in Russia and Eastern Europe. He replied that it would never be practiced in western medicine. "Too radical departure from current ophthalmologic procedures," he asserted. A decade later laser eye surgery became commonplace and relatively safe procedure. This episode indicates medical progress or lack thereof.

Thanks again to Russian researchers, another new eye revolution fast approaches. "Cataract" means waterfall in ancient Greek since patients afflicted with cataract looked through the lenses of their eyes with a blurring of vision similar to looking through a waterfall. The Russian method has been extensively patented in Europe. It uses eye drops containing N-acetyl-carnosine or NAC applied twice daily for an initial period of nine months. Please note that NAC differs chemically from l-carnosine which was mentioned earlier. Both l-carnosine and amino guanidine are good anti-cross linkers and anti-glycators, but *only* l-carnosine with an attached "acetyl" chemical group allows it immediate passage in and out of the fluid of the lenses of the eyes. My own experiences with NAC have pleased me immensely. It gave me renewed hope and encouragement in the medical specialty of anti-aging medicine, and I think you will feel the same way after reading the following tale.

Six years ago, Kaiser Permanente eye specialists diagnosed me as a candidate for cataract surgery within five years. Such are the ravages of aging, I surmised. I also realized that all my strong antioxidants did not reach the lenses of my eyes since they lack blood vessel support. After a tip from my good friend, pharmacist Phil Micans, I began using NAC drops once daily. After three months I experienced no apparent change in my vision. I readily admit my hasty mistake. Then my driver's license came up for renewal, and as a senior I forced myself to visit an ophthalmologist for a routine examination and a letter to the Department of Motor Vehicles. Surprisingly, my left eye had improved from 50 to 25 over 20 and my right eye from 200 to 125. Another nine months of NAC eye drops, and I became eager for another test. My right eye improved from 125 to 70 and my left eye from 25 to 20 over 20. In addition both my intra-ocular pressure and astigmatism showed improvement. Still another nine months, and my right eye had improved to 50 and my left eye to 15 over 20 – namely better vision than normal. After these tests, I jumped for joy. Imagine regaining eyesight that had been fading since my youth. The ravages of aging seemingly reversed themselves. Another nine months elapsed. My left eye had improved further to 10 over 20 and my right eye to 45. My astigmatism improved to the point where I received a new diagnosis of only having slightly astigmatic eyes with an improved intra-ocular pressure reading of 14 on a scale of 9 to 20. That is right; I discovered much to my astonishment that my left eye could read distant street signs better than my younger friends. Also I found myself reading price tags and debit-card terminals without needing glasses. No kidding. I joked with middle-aged friends that I am catching up with them and may even surpass them in physical fitness after another decade of anti-aging treatment.

Then my right eye improved to such an extent that I could obtain a driver's license with this eye alone in the event of a damaged good eye. Since birth my right eye could only read the big "E" on the eye chart. Then, fifty years later I could read five lines down on the eye chart. If there ever was a miracle outside of the Bible, this was it!

Initially, many of my friends and family refused to believe me. They accepted my wild exclamations as the ravings of a mad scientist. Finally, they surrendered to my enthusiasms and began to read for themselves about the Russian miracle of NAC. I have studied and analyzed this subject and would like to report to you the following results of my focused thinking.

A Scientific Explanation for Lens Repair

Scientifically speaking, the eye and other organs are bombarded daily by cascades of free radicals. These radicals react chemically in the lenses of the eye to a form of cross-linking of protein and sugars. These cross linkings originate from semi-permanent chemical bonds between the sugars and the amino groups of proteins in the eye lenses. As described, this gradual biological process is called glycation or cross linking.

N-acetyl carnosine or NAC contains an acetyl group which allows it to become more lipophilic or fat loving which is absorbed by fatty tissues, such as cell membranes.

At slightly acidic pH, this lipophilic molecule can easily transport itself across the membrane of the lens and into its amorphous interior. Once inside, the amino group on the NAC molecule attacks nucleophilically. (Organic-chemistry term used to determine reactivities of various organic molecules.) The byproducts of this reaction pass through the membrane and wash out of the eye with normal tears. As the cross links progressively break open, the waterfall curtain of the cataract gradually disappears and clear sight becomes restored. In my case clear sight in my right eye means better vision than I had at birth. I do not know exactly all the whys and wherefores. I do know that my mother drank while pregnant with me, and alcohol can be tetragenic or causing birth defects.

All of the American ophthalmologists that I have spoken with have read the Russian NAC scientific literature. They find it encouraging, and they await FDA approval which may take many, many years. Does anyone have an extra fifty million dollars lying around in order to move the approval process forward? I suspect that approval lies in the distant future since the economic interests of laser eye surgery are at stake. Further information is available in *"The Cataract Cure"*, 2005, iUniverse, Marios Kyriazis, M.D.

Forget "life, liberty, and the pursuit of happiness". Special interest groups such as Washington lobbyists often determine what is permitted in this country, and therefore as mentioned earlier, special anti-aging supplements such as centrophenoxine and Piracetam are available in Europe and not in the US. The latest lobbying effort seeks to stop small compounding pharmacies from making needed specialty medicines, especially for children, and replace their activities with the drugs of Big Pharma. We really need to demand changes from our government if we expect future benefits of health and longevity. Or we can choose to move abroad where lobbyists hold little political sway.

Renewable Hearing and Preventable Hearing Loss
A team of researchers in New York have reported that patients with severe hearing loss had half as much aldosterone compared to people with normal hearing.

As mentioned in the case study at the start of this chapter, hearing loss has become all too common in today's world since any loud sound over 90 decibels has the long-term effect of damaging our hearing. In general, many people remain unaware of the damage caused by loud noises. If aware, they would press congress to pass laws demanding mufflers on all two-cycle motors in the USA. Is this the third world or what? Many times when walking, my hearing becomes blasted by the unmuffled sound of lawn-cutting equipment. Alternatively, when I am nicely dressed in a shopping center and the noise becomes so unbearable that a normal conversation remains impossible since cleaning crews busy themselves with unmuffled machines. I can well imagine that when these gardeners and cleaners reach their elderly years, many will become hearing impaired.

Consider the fact that young people wear special audio head gear sold without industry or government restrictions regarding maximum decibel levels. It seems that anything goes and who really cares about hearing damage? I do, but in my youth I remember having delusions about living forever. Then, when I reached my thirties —the realities of aging hit me squarely. Considering all the unregulated hearing damage, perhaps this country will become the one with the deaf and dumb leading the blind. Enough about Iraq!

Preventing Hearing Loss
Protect yourself with Peltor ear gear and arrive at your final destination a bit more alert and refreshed.

I know of four solutions for preventing hearing loss. First, wear protective ear plugs and other hearing gear whenever practical. Second, consume 20 mg daily of *vinpocetine*. This will increase blood flow to your damaged hearing centers which in some cases leads to some restored hearing. Alternatively, consume 250 mg daily of *centrophenoxine* or *DMAE* which also improves blood flow and helps the potassium to sodium ratio necessary for proper nerve transmission and hearing. Fourth, and most important of all, have your levels of growth hormone and sex hormones checked. But of course, my *best remedy* employs 125 micrograms of aldosterone twice daily as an effective remedy for adult onset hearing loss. Figure One demonstrates a 33% increase in adult-onset hearing loss. However, do not use these remedies if you have hypertension.

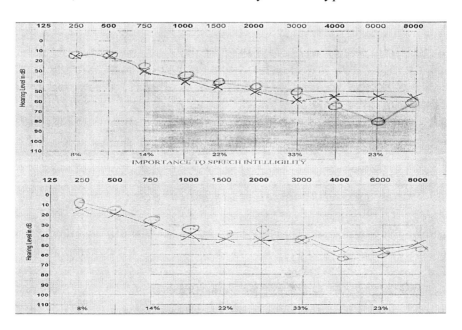

Figure One. Top audiograph before consuming aldosterone. Bottom audiograph where 500 micrograms of aldosterone was taken orally and hearing improved up to 33% at some wavelengths, but only in those with *adult-onset hearing loss* (hearing loss as a result of aging and not from loud noises caused from one's occupation).

Tired of the loud droning sound of jet aircraft while traveling? Forget the $300 electronic noise-canceling ear phones. Try buying a 20 dollar pair of Peltor twin-cup hearing protectors from your local building supply store. Heavy machine operators use this wonderful product for preventing damaged hearing. Peltor's best models will lower noise a *full 50 decibels* which compares favorably to the standard foam ear plugs that only lower noise by 20 decibels. Flight attendants will not like you using them on takeoffs and landings since they hinder *valuable* announcements from the captain and flight crew – something about FAA rules. Should not some rules be violated sometimes in order to protect our health? On the exterior of an aircraft, jet engines emit about 120 decibels of noise, and the inside of the cabin dampens some of it due to insulation. But do not expect it. Peltor gear merely blocks out sounds mechanically to a limit of 50 decibels – no fancy electronics here. Thus people exterior to an airplane work in an environment of 120 minus50 which equals 70 decibels, and this is an acceptable level for preserving good hearing. Protect yourself with Peltor ear gear and arrive at your final destination a bit more alert and refreshed. It works.

Renewable Teeth
I prefer to use animal replacement crowns if one requires teeth with a useful lifespan of at least 100 years or more.

Replacement teeth typically last 10 to 20 years if installed by a competent dentist. Especially short-lived are replacement molars, and dental research has nothing better to offer us at present. I have discussed this problem with industry reps at ADA meetings (American Dental Association), and I have nothing to report. If they are honest with you, many dentists will admit that gold crowns on molars last longer than porcelain or plastic ones since they tolerate a grinding pressure of only a few thousand pounds per square inch or *psi*. Gold tolerates higher pressures, but for the ultimate in pressure tolerance, one must look to the animal kingdom. The present-day animal kingdom uses molars similar in size to human molars that will endure 15,000 psi, and during Jurassic periods, T. Rex tolerated molar pressures of approximately 18,000 psi. Also, the amazing teeth of the hyena and the shark allow them to fully devour the carcass of most land and sea animals, bones and everything. Only the viscera remain unchewable due to its rubbery nature. I prefer to use animal replacement crowns if one requires teeth with a useful lifespan of at least 100 years or more. Interestingly, one of our founding fathers, George Washington, used human and animal teeth replacements.

Yes, sir, 15,000 psi pressure tolerance and a perfect crystalline matrix of pure calcium phosphate. If you can source animal replacement molars, then your dentist's local dental lab can shape the bottom of them to fit as crowns over your existing molars. Unfortunately, no synthetic replacement equivalents to animal teeth have become available. Who knows, perhaps "fashionistas" may consider it fashionable to install sharks teeth in their mouths instead of merely wearing them around their necks.

Realistically, I encourage people to wait until Europe develops something better and somehow manages to slip past congressional lobbyists and our FDA. Imagine living into the 22nd century with functioning choppers.

Enhanced Senses In General
Who says dogs have the best noses.

As previously implied, vinpocetine and aldosterone may enhance hearing to such an extent that loud noises become irritating, if not painful. Vinpocetine sells over the counter at some pharmacies in Europe, and the side effects remain minimal. Vinpocetine and aldosterone will also benefit slightly our other senses: The eyes become more sensitive to color, the nose becomes more sensitive to pungent smells, and one's sense of touch improves. In fact, all of your senses can be further enhanced by consuming at bedtime 500 mg of carnosine or N-acetyl carnosine (NAC) and/or 500 mg ornithine/arginine (Twin Labs). Carnosine and its acetyl analogs help to reverse glycation throughout the body just as NAC reverses glycation specifically in the lens of the eyes. Ornithine/arginine mixtures kick start metabolism's *Krebs cycle* which in turn increases biochemical activity throughout your body and especially in your skin. A proof of this increased metabolism in skin is evidenced by the flare up of cold sores in and around the mouth of some people when consuming ornithine/arginine supplements.

Yet another way to enhance the senses is through training. Contrary to popular belief, the human sense of smell is nearly equivalent to canines if one properly trains it. You have read about the "Joys of Menopause." How about the joys of pleasant smells? **The Swedish language even has a special word for pleasant smells as opposed to nasty smells, namely the words "doft" as opposed to "lukt," respectively.** Pleasing smells or "doft" make the human experience worthwhile. Each one of your nostrils contains over two thousand nerve endings – a greater quantity than in any other sense organ in your body. These thousands of nerve endings must have been put there for a purpose, and I contend that it is to detect "doft" and sometimes even "lukt". Interestingly, science has shown that these nerve endings can detect down to *picogram* amounts of pungent substances such as ammonia. A picogram is 1 X 10 to the negative twelfth power, or one millionth of a microgram. Analytical chemists readily admit that such minuscule quantities remain undetectable to their analytical equipment.

Unfortunately, I am unable to train anyone in improving their sense of smell. Short of working for a perfume factory in France or for my friend, Gail Heyman of Giorgio's perfume, I suggest acquiring my pugnacious curiosity and determination in smelling nearly everything you come in contact with, especially gourmet foods, flowers, and perfumes. Also use Zantac® antihistamine since it clears the sinuses quite nicely for better smelling experiences. Enjoy.

Smell Enhancement
For enhancement and quality of life, should not we all try to return partially to our caveman roots and engage our most basic senses?

Nobel Prize winner, Professor Richard Feynman of Cal Tech addressed the issue of the human sense of smell in his book, *"Surely*

You're Joking, Mr. Feynman". He demonstrated his acutely-trained sense of smell to his academic friends as follows. At a house party, he would wear gloves and place a high stack of dusty books in the center of a table. He would leave the room and ask his guests to remove only one book from the stack with their bare hands and replace the book back in the stack. Then he would return to the room and identify the moved book solely with his sense of smell. Feynman smelled hand oil and perspiration from the disturbed book with his trained nose.

A further demonstration of our incredible powers of smell became apparent in the small town of Gras, France. Gras is the perfume capital of the world where tons of flowers grow annually, and their essences extracted for the perfume industry. The perfume industry hires special perfume snifters who identify different perfume smells, or doft, such as floral, woody, alcohol, musty, etc. The most experienced snifters have Charles de Gaulle size-noses and can clearly distinguish over 700 individual smells (doft), and this allows them to blend perfumes and create beautiful aromas. Over 700. Who says dogs have the best noses?

If we would only train ourselves using my brand of pugnacious curiosity, we all could have an incredible sense of smell, and ditto for an acute sense of colors. Personally, I have trained my eyes to detect many subtle shades and mixtures of blues, reds, yellows, and purples that are unfamiliar to even normally non-color blinded people. I did this by badgering three friends of mine with Master of Fine Arts degrees into teaching me to oil paint. I amazed these friends by my unbridled curiosity since the only way I know to acquire a new skill requires getting enthusiastically involved. When one learns to paint as a hobby, new colors and shades present themselves and a new universe of the color spectrum reveals itself. Who says only artists and greenies can enjoy rainbows of color? For example, in the paintings of Bonnard and Matisse, I can see with the naked eye up to seven layers of color in which each layer is translucently laid upon each of the others. Other artists known as *"colorists"* can see what I see but not members of the general public. Possibly our senses become blunted by the fast-paced demands of modern living. For enhancement and quality of life, we should try to return partially to our caveman roots and engage our most basic senses. This would entail training our senses somewhat like the French do and turning off the TV and getting closer to nature again. I made this comment since years ago while engaged to a lovely French girl, and I got to know her, her family and her culture quite well. In my opinion the French can be much more down-to-earth with a genuine curiosity if not obsession for color and doft especially compared to Americans. But perhaps I am prejudiced, or at the very least jaded. Do you think that enhanced sense of color and smell seem worthwhile, or are we already satisfied with what modern life hands us on a platter?

If you really engage your eyes into improving your sense of color, a new vista of experience awaits you. Trust me. For example, if you study post-impressionist art, you will notice that Pablo Picasso was one of the greatest draftsmen of the last century, but in the realm of color, he must have been color blind. Peruse his paintings and drawings and notice his use of an *arbitrary* color pallet. In other words, he chose any old color anywhere without rhyme or reason. He could not distinguish color differences. For this reason Picasso disliked the well-known and highly colorful paintings of Bonnard since to the colorblind, Bonnard's paintings lack clear, linear definition. See for yourself.

Miscellaneous New Body Parts under Development: Renewable Skin and Organs
Eventually Dr. Atala grew in his Petri dishes whole, complete organs such as bladders which were harvested and transplanted into needy patients, much like new mufflers are replaced on your car.

In the pipeline of regeneration tissue research are entire arrays of new body parts which come custom-tailored to your body: urine-processing tissue, insulin-producing tissue, salivary-gland tissue, heart values and repair tissue, penis-repair tissue, vaginal tissue, and new blood vessels and cartilage. The latest research reveals new bladders that were installed in seven children suffering from *spina bifida*. All seven are doing well, and the oldest bladder has functioned for more than six years.

Interestingly, a fully functioning replacement uterus has been developed. At the Wake Forest Research Park, noted researcher Dr.

Anthony Atala refers to himself as the "Man Who Would Cheat Death" – thus, this chapter's title. As a surgeon he harvests primitive, Petri dish bottom-layered cells and grows them in his lab using special growth nutrients and plastic scaffolding for shape – all without stem cells. Instead of stem cells, he only uses fully developed human-bladder cells. Future research hopes to use basic *human stem cells* which would develop into mature bladder cells if only certain religious people in Washington would accept the idea. As a result, stem cell research develops at a fast pace in such remote corners of the globe as Singapore and Korea, despite the positive efforts of the "Govenator," Arnold Schwarzenegger, and the negative efforts of some Washington politicos.

Eventually, Dr. Atala grew in his Petri dishes whole, complete organs such as bladders which were harvested and transplanted into needy patients, much like new mufflers are replaced on your car. Great.

Teflon Skin and Membranes
Skin becomes impervious to bacteria, virus and chemical attack.

The remainder of this chapter speculates on possible future enhancements that do not exist today. I will now speculate as to what *might* happen in the near future in contrast to the rest of this book, which only addresses hard scientific facts. Please bear with my fantasies.

I have long fantasized about the possibility of enhancing the human body. In science fiction people like the "Bionic Woman" are outfitted with special prosthetics for increased speed and agility. I realize these prospects are a long way from reality, but I have my habits as an adventurous yet responsible scientist. If I did not speculate about the possibilities of the future, there would be no future, only the orthodox and status quo. Which would you prefer?

Think if skin, organs, and membranes could improve their resistance to extreme heat, cold, and radiation. For example, in an extreme desert environment, survival means preventing dehydration and not cooling the body. Retaining bodily fluids in a hot climate is essential for both health and survival. At the other extreme, a freezing cold climate means keeping both the body's core and extremities at temperatures above 90 degrees F. Extreme cold forces the body to warm its core which allows the extremities to freeze. Frostbite results.

A third climate protection would be increased resistance to solar radiation. The sun dries and ages the skin which eventually leads to collagen cross-linking and various skin cancers, e.g. melanomas. Think if your skin and entire body were more resistant to extreme heat, cold and sun. In coming decades we may well need this technology with the depletion of the ozone layers and the melting of the polar caps.

Since the late seventies, I have investigated the possibility of enhancing skin and its resistance to cold, heat, and free radicals *at the molecular level*. Mother Nature already enhances skin and membranes in animals called *"extremophiles."* For example, *thermophile* microbes can withstand temperatures of 238 degrees Fahrenheit since they possess stiffening agents in their membranes to keep them from melting away. At the other extreme, extremophiles such as *fridgophile* bacteria thrive in the high Andes mountains since their membranes are "loosey-goosey" or very fluid and amorphous (gelatin-like) which resists stiffening and freezing climates.

In the future, I envision human membranes and skin slowly and gradually replaced with special types of polyunsaturated fatty acids, or PUFAs. PUFAs normally provide stiffening and flexibility to skin, and my specially synthesized PUFAs contain fluorine atoms instead of hydrogen. Note that elemental fluorine is probably bad for your teeth, but perhaps it would improve your skin. I would like to propose some practical benefits of fluorinated PUFAs as follows.

- Walk about in the ozone-poor Australian sun without being covered with heavy clothing or sun screen.
- Skin becomes impervious to bacteria, virus and chemical attack.
- Cells and their sensitive mitochondria resist oxidation, peroxidation, free radicals and aging which causes a boom in medical research such as bionic living-organisms and their bionic cells and membranes used as test models for curing many major diseases.

I realize all this is a dream of the future. The DuPont website offers Teflon® fluoro polymers as "solutions for your engineering design needs". I am with them. Let us go for it. But a dream is technically possible only if financial support becomes available. Got a few hundred million bucks lying around, and you do not know what to do with it? Join the polyfluoro future.

All scientifically inclined readers please read more details about my fluoridated skin in appendix E.

Future Speculations:
Renew Your Old Body for a Young One
"If the Devil had shown up at my house, instead of calling on dreary Faust, and offered me a perfectly functioning body until death in exchange for my soul, I'd had said, it's a deal bud, with joy." Martha Gellhorn, famous 20ᵗʰ century journalist.

I would like to speculate long into the future. Twenty years from now it might be technically possible *to exchange* one's aging body for a healthy, muscular, youthful one. This will raise moral objections and will seem distasteful to many people, including me.

But the new body technology is right around the corner, thanks to fund-raising efforts of celebrities such as the late quadriplegic Christopher Reeves and others who have raised millions for research that repairs the neurons of the spinal cord damaged or severed through accidents. *This intensive, ongoing research may eventually yield the discovery of a growth factor that will promote neurons to reconnect with one another.* Despite intensive worldwide research, *human* growth factors are unknown as of 2008, but they do exist in a wide range of other rather *primitive* creatures such as salamanders, zebra fish, deer (antlers), spiders, starfish and sea cucumbers. See the appendix. At a rate of two centimeters daily these animals simply regenerate themselves using their own growth factors and distinct stem-like cells. One recent significant finding originated from the lab of Dr. Mark Keating who identified a gene for the re-growth of *blastemas* (a stem cell source) called the *fgf 20 gene* in Zebra fish and comparable to the *hsp 60 gene* in humans. These and other underlying genetic mechanisms remain largely unknown. I am not a specialist in genetics; therefore I have no opinions as to how one could leap forward with advances here, especially without adequate support from Washington.

Welcome to the brave new world of re-growing on your own. If and when this stem-cell re-growth becomes possible in humans, a new body tech industry will develop. In the meantime the government should permit organ transplants from the 50,000 Americans who die yearly in auto accidents. Think if only those *refusing* to donate their organs were so marked on their driver's licenses instead of the contrary? In other words, everyone not refusing would automatically become a donor candidate when they pass their driver's test. After all, driving is a privilege and not a God-given right. Ditto for the availability of organs.

There is an acute shortage of transplant organs in Hawaii due to the refusal of some ethnic groups (Philippinos, for example) to allow donations due to their religious beliefs. The lives of the suffering and dying should take precedence over religious beliefs, both in Hawaii and in North America.

Whole Body Transplant
"I saw the hideous phantasm of a man stretched out, and then, on the working of some powerful engine, show signs of life and stir with an uneasy, half-vital motion . . . . .He sleeps; but he is awakened; he opens his eyes." Frankenstein by Mary Shelley London, 1818

In coming decades whole body transplants will become technically possible. Many asked me not to explain this technology further because of its somewhat ghoulish and politically incorrect nature. Suffice it to say that it will happen using today's commonplace vascular surgical techniques and organ tissue typing combined with future advances in re-connecting severed spinal cords. Christopher Reeves would have approved while many others would reject it by labeling it as "Frankenstein". This situation reminds me of the French labeling bio-engineered American seeds for grain crops as "Franken-foods". Perhaps so. All this persuades me to ask if America anticipates being at the forefront of science and medical technology in the 21st century? I have my doubts.

The end of this chapter speculates about the future, and therefore departs a bit from the solid science of the preceding chapters. I would like to remind the reader that I would never have envisioned and carried-through with the inventions and developments of the first seven chapters if I did not often try to think outside the box and into the future. Perhaps I have a bad habit of asking the why's and how's instead of asking the politically correct, appropriate, and orthodox. To paraphrase Helen Keller, "The subversive of today becomes the orthodox of tomorrow".

Recommendations

- Find an anti-aging health care professional.
- For the adventurous: Partner with the above for hormone adjustment back to youthful values of people in their thirties.
- Replace teeth with the best possible materials.
- Use Can C eye drops (l-acetyl carnitine) twice daily for 2 years.
- Consume 250 mg centrophenoxine or 40 mg vinpocetine for enhanced hearing. For hearing loss and jet lag take 125 mcg twice daily *aldosterone*.
- Use Peltor twin-cup hearing protectors.
- For enhanced senses in general: Consume min. 250 mg daily carnosine caps.
- Consume minimum 500 mg daily ornithine/arginine caps.
- Practice Professor Feynman's sense of smell exercises.
- Support medical research, especially Christopher Reeve's project for spinal cord growth factors.
- Eat fresh, raw or semi-raw fish, fruit, nuts, and vegetables daily along with Vitamins B-6, B-12 and folic acid.

Golden keys to longevity #8

- *After middle age, enhance the senses by judicious daily use of l-carnosine capsules for the body, l-acetyl-carnosine drops for the eyes, and aldosterone for the hearing and nocturia.*

161

Appendix E: A Fluoridated Skin Proposal for the Future
Our skin would become chemical and free-radical resistant.

Our skin and cell membranes are structured primarily of polyunsaturated fatty acids or *PUFAs*. PUFAs are mostly composed of palmitic, linoleic, linolenic, and arachidonic acids composed of 16 to 23 carbon atoms linked together in a string. The end of the string contains an acid group, symbol -COOH, and the other end, a methyl group, symbol -CH3. Along the string itself, most carbon atoms surround themselves with two hydrogen atoms, symbol -CH2- , with the exceptions of one or more double carbon-carbon bonds such as -HC=CH- . As previously explained, these unsaturated double bonds become highly susceptible to chemical, radiation and free-radical attack. When this occurs, PUFAs become damaged and if part of a cell membrane, the membrane then becomes damaged and the cell dies.

I proposed replacement of many of the hydrogen atoms in PUFAs with fluorine atoms. I name these new substance polyfluoro-PUFAs. If I replace many of the normal PUFAs in the body with polyfluoro-PUFAs, many interesting enhancements would occur as displayed in Figure 1.

Since polyfluoro-PUFAs are similar chemically to the Dupont polymer, Teflon®, the body would become more Teflon-like. The skin would become more silky-smooth, slippery, and resist heat and oil much like your Teflon-coated frying pan. The double bonds of the polyfluoro-PUFAs would increase their resistance to solar and even nuclear radiation. Consequently, they and our skin would become chemical and free-radical resistant. In fact, the only way Teflon materials bond or stick to themselves are melting them slightly with an extremely powerful organic acid called *HF* for hydrofluoric acid.

Chapter 9
A New Twist on Skin

Make It Renewable and Elastic
"There's a Playboy edition you don't want to miss: Girls of the AARP. One sign you may not be pinup material – you yourself have centerfolds." Bill Maher

Ms. S, age 48, had an allergic reaction to a new skin care line which resulted in a few small bumps. She had hoped that it would disappear on its own, but she was sadly mistaken. She visited numerous dermatologists who prescribed several remedies including the drug, *Diprolene®*, but her face became even worse. She now had horrible red and discolored skin patches that extended down the sides of her nose and across her chin. One dermatologist asked her if she thought she might have *rosacea, a* common condition in the aging skin of the face. She answered that she never had any skin problems until she used prescription drugs.

The poor little miss. She continued from bad to worse with treatments that experimented with antibiotics, sulfa lotions, and special skin cleaners. She arrived at her appointment with a strained appearance and disheveled clothing after months of worry. After several sleepless nights, her cortisol was elevated which was evident by dark circles under her eyes and splotches of large and small inflamed bumps on her cheeks. Her neck muscles were tense. She even refrained from looking in a mirror since the tender red bumps had traveled from her face, down her neck, and onto her chest. At times her skin felt sunburned and chapped. She was beside herself with anxiety and implored immediate help.

In a staccato, strained voice, Ms. S asked whether Liquid Silver 400 PPM formula might help to heal the infected bumps. She also asked if she dare start a nutritional program consisting of folic acid, Vitamin E, zinc, evening primrose oil (GLA), and multiple vitamin supplements. Later, in a near whisper, she blurted out that she had recently entered menopause and quit smoking. She needed positive solutions in a hurry after many unrewarding visits to less knowledgeable physicians.

Unfortunately her skin condition seemed like rosacea, but not caused by her medications or new cosmetics. No one really knows what causes rosacea, and there is no known treatment that worked well on everyone. With no clear and standard medical response to her affliction, she tried several treatments in the hope of alleviating her problem. With kind understanding, I recommended Silver 400 PPM formula applied twice daily. Rosacea seems to worsen with hormone shifts attributed to menopause, and therefore, she should first address her hormone problems, especially the stress hormone, cortisol. Secondly, *hyperbaric oxygen treatment* was recommended which has shown some effectiveness with rosacea. She may even want to attempt MSM treatment from vrp.com. If her skin had been infected, mastic gum treatment using Cease Fire™ would have proven effective in eliminating gastric and dermal bacteria. Finally, with great empathy and understanding she was encouraged to check the internet for rosacea support groups that could help her further with still other alternative therapies for this difficult-to-treat condition.

I would also like to add that Ms. S should have a *comprehensive* hormone analysis of dozens of hormones *only* available at meridianvalleylab.com. At her age and with her entering menopause, she will surely need several unbalanced hormones. I also believe that she should consume weekly at least 30,000 IU of Vitamin D3, a vital skin vitamin often lacking even in those who live in sunny climes. She might also switch to *Cover Girl Makeup* since I have noticed that it performs better from a hypoallergenic viewpoint than its competitors.

Living in Our Skin and Broadening Our Horizons
I have also combined this knowledge with recent advances in measurement of hormones.

Think if we could widen our horizons in regard to our understanding of human skin. Dermatologists have extensively studied it from a narrow disease viewpoint while the cosmetic industry exploits it from a narrow profit viewpoint. In this chapter I have attempted to explore human skin with an anti-aging approach. I have attempted to bridge together the knowledge of dermatologists with chemists, free-radical physicists, and anthropologists -- a multidisciplinary application. I have also combined this knowledge with recent advances in measurement of hormones as reflected in my advice to Ms. S.

Living in Your Skin, Historically
Longevity increased by the additional detoxifying effect of a third kidney.

Anthropologists teach that human skin has evolved from hairy, non-sweating proto-humans/apes to modern humans, who are rather hairless but have enormous numbers of sweat and oil glands. Apparently human evolution took off two million years ago when primates, who could no longer be called apes, appeared in the savannahs of East Africa. These early humans ran long distances in open fields, and they needed to cool and detoxify their brains and bodies with additional sweat and oil glands. Early humans evolved an enormous number of sweat and oil glands for those purposes, which in turn permitted their brains to expand and their longevity to increase. Furthermore, brains expanded from the cooling effect of sweat evaporation, and longevity increased by the additional detoxifying effect of a *third kidney*, namely enormous numbers of oil glands rapidly eliminating oil-soluble toxins. Increases in longevity and brain size allowed increased planning and hunting which consequently resulted in an increased use of tools and traveling over the entire African continent. Humans began appearing in Central Asia at this time.

Human skin was also extremely accommodating to changes in radiation from the sun. Heavy solar radiation promoted an increase in *melanocytes* (pigmented cells) which produced *melanin*, a darkening pigment plentiful in humans from sunny climes. In addition, melanin granules developed in *keratinocytes* (cells with hardened membranes) as a response to tanning. Low solar radiation retarded melatonin and light-skinned humans appeared in cloudy climes. Those humans who migrated from one clime to another easily adapted their skin to their new environments. This adaptation allowed for increases in longevity since skin cancers such as melanoma could be minimized with readily adaptable melanocytes. But this adaptation was not perfect, and those fair-skinned humans who persisted with heavy sun bathing in sunny climes paid the price of mutant (changing) melanocytes, skin cancer, and shortened life spans. Fortunately, these effects were somewhat ameliorated by a tumor suppressor and transcription factor called *p53* which served as a protector of DNA in multicellular organisms for the past half a billion years. In more recent times from the Renaissance to the 1940's, humans have also protected themselves by covering up and avoiding sun exposure.

Human skin had other vital functions. Tattooing or painting the skin helps humans to attract mates. For example, woman painted around their eyes with the message, "Look at me, I am attractive", and men body painted themselves with the message announcing their warrior prowess and potential as a mate.

Still another function of human skin was an abundance of sensory glands that detect heat, cold, and sense of touch. Mother Nature has shaped these glands like onions, and they are ubiquitous throughout the human skin organ. They also function in controlling body temperature, eliminating waste (a third kidney), producing Vitamin D, and providing the body with an outer barrier. Contrary to popular belief, the skin remains unaffected *permanently* by coffee, smoking, rich food, dirt, dust, make-up, lack of sleep, or lack of exercise.

The Sun: Your Skin's Worst Enemy
Another method for increasing exposure to the sun by about 40 minutes uses EDTA bath salts which chelate or remove iron and other heavy metals from the skin.

The skin becomes drastically damaged from many years of excessive sun. Ask anyone from Australia where up to 60% of the older population has AK (*actinic keratosis*), a hardening and *cross linking* of the skin which sometimes progresses to *squamous cell* carcinoma (SCC). When diehard sun worshippers reach the ripe age of 34 to 38 years, their skin has greater difficulty repairing itself. Facial skin becomes more leathery in texture, especially those with fair complexions. The sun accelerates aging in the skin and may lead to life-threatening melanomas. In sunny climates, fair-skinned people over 40 who have been sun lovers for several decades have experienced a near-epidemic of skin cancer on the ears and nose. In fact, one million new cases were diagnosed last year in the US. These cancers are easily removed, but only one single melanoma cell can and does migrate to other areas in the body and initiate cancer tumors. This has been the case with my father, Frank; whereas his father avoided the sun at all costs.

A real breakthrough has occurred in the treatment of the most common skin cancers. The new treatment uses a topical cream called "*BEC-5*" which shows 100% efficiency in removing non-melanoma BCC (*basal cell carcinoma*) and SCC. www.antiaging-motivate.com. I have tried it on keratosis-hardened skin and found that it provides relief with a slight tingling sensation.

At the other extreme in climates, the Swedish sun shines brightly during summers only. Consequently, most Swedes do not get skin cancer unless they burn their skins abroad or use solar beds. Avoidance of the sun seems like the best policy, and has in fact been the standard historical practice in America and Europe for hundreds of years until modern times. Your grandparents and those before them knew that sun exposure was unfashionable and unwarranted.

The fashion of by-gone years encouraged lily white skins. Too bad we cannot readily adopt the long-lost habits of our ancestors.

If you really must tan yourself, I heartily recommend the self-tanning cream from Estée Lauder called "*Self-Sun*". This provides you with a natural looking tan and even hides some unaesthetic skin blemishes. While not using this excellent cream, I try to cover up as much as possible with clothing such as long-sleeve shirts, sun hats, etc. For a moisturizer I always use natural hyaluronic acid cream applied to exposed areas one daily. I also try to use a heavy PABA blocking cream while on the beach or working in the garden. These blocking creams are only about 95% effective in blocking solar radiation. To my knowledge, the only cream that blocks 100% is *zinc oxide ointment* which is critical for participating in water and boating sports. As mentioned earlier, another method for increasing exposure to the sun by about 40 minutes uses EDTA bath salts which chelate or remove iron and other heavy metals from the skin. This bathing ritual eliminates heavy metal catalysts which promote free-radical cascades when sunlight irradiates the skin. I favor this valuable chelating bath-salt method, especially if one lives in a sunny clime. Also, I believe that Ms. S's rosacea may benefit from facial washes with EDTA.

What Causes Skin Imperfections?
The acid mantle remains essential for skin health, integrity, and resistance to bacteria and virus.

The skin has two important groups of glands. Dermatologists classify the first group as sweat glands which include the *apocrine* and *eccrine* glands. Bacteria work at the openings of the sweat glands and give sweat its distinctive odor. A second group is *the sebaceous glands* that are especially numerous on the face and scalp. The sebaceous glands open upon the base of all hair follicles (Figure 1). They lubricate the hair and prevent the skin from drying-out through their secretion of sebum. Sebum contains over forty different organic alcohols, acids and esters that continually cover skin and hair with an oily protective coating. Scientists call this coating the *acid mantle* since it has an acidic pH of about 5. The acid mantle remains essential for skin health, integrity, and resistance to bacteria and viruses. Therefore, washing too frequently with soap may in fact expose you to more bacteria.

Unfortunately, in many people the sebaceous glands remain sensitive to varying levels of sex hormones. For example, excess testosterone in men and excess androgen in both genders may cause cells at the mouth of the sebaceous glands to multiply rapidly and increase in size. This effect causes sebum stoppage. Bacteria attack this bottled-up sebum and cause inflammation that we call acne. Washing the skin with rubbing alcohol and treating it with retinoic acid eliminates much of this problem, but my favorite method employs 50,000 units of Vitamin A daily for two weeks followed by two weeks abstinence. Indeed, men can alleviate baldness by applying and washing twice daily with "*Tween 80*" or "*Polysorb 80*" as the Germans have used for decades (available at vrp.com). These soap-like liquids penetrate the scalp and hair follicles, combine with sebum oils, and aid sebum in removing it from the body. Also, another treatment for men only is consuming 0.5 mg weekly of *Avodart*^{TM} which effectively blocks 93% of the scalp's testosterone from converting into the hormone *dihydrotestosterone* (DHT). DHT kills hair follicles. For both men and women, *Minoxidil*^{TM} has become another treatment for hair loss since it dilates the blood vessels of hair follicles and allows more oxygen and nutrients that are helpful in follicle growth and function. Still a third method employs 30 mg daily of the natural hormone progesterone applied vigorously to the scalp to block excessive DHT.

Skin Wrinkling
I would go easy on the transition metals (copper and manganese) with the large "d" orbitals that can readily receive and give off electrons which form damaging free radicals.

During the last thirty years, scientists have begun to understand how, where and why skin wrinkles. The "aging clock" controlling wrinkling skin can be slowed but not stopped by anti-aging nutrients. Probably the best direct and immediate method for eliminating existing wrinkles is dermabrasion. Dermabrasion lightly scrapes the skin by using a small sanding wheel. This method proves itself more effective than chemical peeling since the skin heals faster and more evenly.

A second method uses a variety of fillers such as hyaluronic acid from roosters. Beverly Hills physician Dr. Arnold Klein strongly advocates the fillers *Restylane®* and *Botox®* even though they have short lives of only a few months. They will fill deep facial *rhytids* or grooves. The FDA has recently approved a more long-term filler *Artefill®* which is made from bonding sterilized calf collagen to microscopic plastic beads. I have my reservations about its use until many years of experience prove its value.

A third method uses conventional plastic surgery to pull the skin tighter. A fourth method is the focus of anti-aging research.

Enter the eminent dermatologist, Dr. Perricone, and his "thymic peptides". Dr. Perricone states flatly that wrinkles are tiny wounds, and they may be treated by decreasing inflammation, releasing growth hormone, and increasing production of collagen, elastin, and blood vessels. His thymic peptides supplements achieve exactly what he promises. www.vrp.com He also advises liberal use of Vitamins B-5, C, copper, zinc, magnesium and manganese, all of which aid in repair of tissue damage. I believe it, but I would go easy on the transition metals (copper and manganese) with the large "d" orbitals that can readily receive and give off electrons which form damaging free radicals. Large "d" orbitals are mostly found in transition and other metals which allows them to easily conduct electricity as well as become catalysts for free-radical reactions.

Another example of the ill effects of free radicals I call free-radical burn. For those over the age of forty-five, the skin becomes dry and discolored and wrinkled and scientifically, cross-linked. Free radicals combined with poor hormone balance – such as high cortisol (hypoadrenalism) -- have literally burned the skin and its underlying mitochondria with significant losses of function and appearance. And *the skin organ reflects the condition and appearance of organs throughout the body.* The ravages of this aging effect can only be slowed at present with multiple daily doses of *strong* antioxidants, free-radical scavengers, chelators, and the best of all hormone creams, testosterone for men and estradiol for women. Smooth, youthful-appearing skin will be your reward.

The following figure illustrates some of the underlying chemistry and mechanics of aging skin, and it reveals the chemical and mechanical nature of collagen.

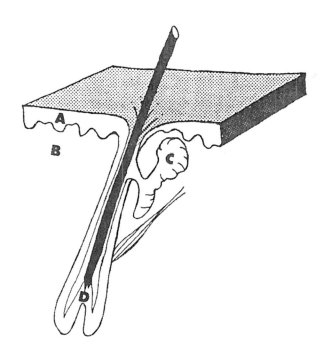

In Figure One, the outermost layer of skin is called the epidermis. Under this is the skin's largest layer called the dermis. The dermis contains a structural substance called collagen which is made from stringy bundles of parallel fibers which give our skin pliability and elasticity.

Get That Glow of Youth Look Back into Your Skin and Eyes
Thus, T3 has become especially valuable for men and women experiencing hair loss as they age.

Dr. Perricone and his thymic peptides provide an excellent solution for skin care, but I would like to propose a more permanent solution. Have you ever wondered why young people have a special sparkle to their eyes and a fresh, blushing rosiness to their cheeks? I have. And I have decided to do something about it. Through constant experimenting and implementing my multidisciplinary research method, I have devised the following protocol.

For those over the age of 40, try rubbing into your facial skin 5 mg of topical testosterone cream. Add to that 30 mg of a bio-identical progesterone cream. When these critical hormones are deficient, facial and hand skin become slack and inelastic. For even more dramatic effect, treat the above with 10 mg T3 thyroid hormone. But tread carefully here since if you apply T3 to hair follicles, hair growth will dramatically begin, and ensuing medical condition called "*hirsutism*" (excessive hair growth) may be experienced. These two wonderful hormones have become especially valuable for men and women experiencing hair loss as they age.

The above topical cream formulation will yield a fresh, youthful glow, and this effect has nothing to do with the usual cosmetic-ad hype that has hijacked these words. With these remedies you will achieve a freshness and glow of many teenagers, and all without masking your appearance behind cosmetics.

A Solution for Itching Skin
A valuable treatment for any nerve disorder that has become bothersome.

Mrs. W asked him if she should take progesterone (*HerBalance™)* cream with the hormone, pregnenolone and pregnenolone capsules (30 mg) at the same time. Also, she asked what dosages he recommends. Mrs. W had chronic skin itching problems, and she found that these two products often helped her. Before employing these two products, she was distraught from constant itching day and night without relief. Furthermore, she exclaimed that pregnenolone has totally changed her life since her depression has vanished.

She could combine the HerBalance cream with pregnenolone and pregnenolone capsules. Since the dosage requirement is different for different people, 10, 30, and 100 mg capsules were recommended for her. For itchy skin, she might also try *Lithium Orotate* 1-2 capsules twice daily, but not for long term use. This is a great nerve stabilizer, and it may help to further alleviate her itching. Lithium is a valuable temporary treatment for any nerve disorder that has become bothersome. Lithium Orotate from vrp.com truly helps in reducing skin itching.

Scientific Explanation

Why Is Collagen Elastic and Pliable?
This biochemical effect gives elasticity to the skin and arteries and can be viewed in the elderly when dehydrated.

The individual fibers in collagen's stringy bundles are linked together by a special chemical bond. During the last thirty years, Dr. A.J. Bailey in England and others have discovered the location, nature and mechanism of these special bonds.

During the growth phase of mammals, these bonds are easily split and reformed, split and reformed, over and over again. This reversible characteristic provides the fibers with their elasticity since this splitting and reforming allows individual fibers to smoothly glide next to one another. The fibers are loose and pliable when the bonds split, and rigid when the bonds become reformed as depicted in Figure 2.

Figure Two. Two collagen fibers (R and R') lying adjacent to each other owe their elasticity to reversible chemical bonds. These bonds are separate and open (-CHO and HN-) at the top of this drawing, and together and closed (wide arrow) at the bottom of this figure. The opening and closing of these bonds allows the fibers to glide freely and to remain rigid relative to each other. This reversible opening and closing is caused by the uptake and shedding of water (H2O) which hydrates and dehydrates the skin, respectively. This biochemical effect gives elasticity to the skin and arteries and can be viewed in the elderly when dehydrated. During temporary hydration, the skin becomes less elastic. This can be demonstrated by pinching and releasing the skin on the back of the hand.

However, during the mammal aging more and more of the reformed bonds become irreversibly rigid. In Figure Two above, the slow life-long process depicts this rigidity. Scientists suspect that oxidation causes it. Antioxidant and other nutrients will delay somewhat this oxidation with the help of the Vitamin B-1 derivative, *benfotiamine* (Milgamma). Also, *carnosine* helps to reverse it somewhat and a minimum 250 mg daily should be consumed if one wishes to minimize skin wrinkling.

The effective nutrient, benfotiamine prevents nerve cell and blood vessel damage caused by excessive amounts of sugar building up in the tissues. Benfotiamine also helps to prevent glycation or cross-linking in the skin and collagen fibers. It has a method of action similar to carnosine.

Still another method for preventing and reversing skin sagging, tissue connectivity, fat-pad volume, and denting of cheeks and temples (concavity) employs the frequent use of human growth hormone and other deficient hormones.

The Miracle of Carnosine
Carnosine is a vital key to any anti-aging regimen that seeks to prevent deterioration from aging and the pre-diseases.

Carnosine is an amazing molecule composed of two amino acids (*dipeptide of alanine* and *histamine*) bonded together much like the two amino acids that bind together the common sweetener, *aspartame* (NutraSweet). The muscles, brain, and lenses of the eyes already contain high concentrations of it. Apparently, when concentrations falter during aging, cataracts develop in the lenses of the eyes, and muscles stiffen throughout the body. The *misfolding of proteins* causes muscle stiffening, and carnosine has the task of effectively repairing this damage. Since protein damage becomes common in such diseases as Alzheimer's and mad cow disease, it likely shares responsibility for many other diseases described in previous chapters. Carnosine remains a true *protective dipeptide* since it prevents high blood pressure, excess copper and zinc, free-radical catalysts, damaged proteins, lack of antioxidant and enzymatic lines of defense, Alzheimer's plaques and neuronal tangles, stroke, slow wound healing, muscle fatigue and glycation of the lenses of the eyes. Figures 2 and 3 depict two beneficial mechanisms of carnosine.

Obviously carnosine is a vital key to any anti-aging regimen that seeks to prevent deterioration from aging and adult-onset problems. Serious anti-aging programs would include 250 to 1,000 mg daily of carnosine taken on an empty stomach or in combination with other chelators and anti-glycators. I also combine *hyaluronic acid* capsules, 6 daily, to my cocktail. Hyaluronic acid lotion may also be applied to exposed skin areas to further moisturized it and make skin shinny. This combination I call my skin anti-aging cocktail. Large doses of 500 mg carnosine may be taken in the evenings. My cocktail works in conjunction with other catabolic (breakdown) processes occurring naturally during the sleep cycle.

The enormous benefits of carnosine remain unrecognized in the USA. For example, older cardiac patients become amazed by the results when using it and measuring the effects with an instrument called a *"Cardiotrack"*. Using this instrument some patients' reflective index fell from 81% to 42% using carnosine. (Index of relative flexibility of one's arteries.) This means that older patients nearly double their muscle and arterial flexibility. Thus, flexibility doubled! Similar improvements were also found in older patients' skin. Carnosine and hyaluronic acid therapy works.

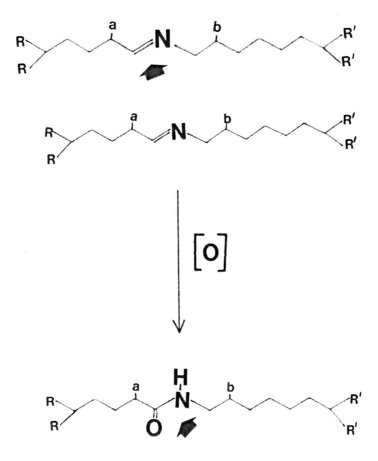

Figure 3. Humans stop growing and maturing between 20 to 30 years of age. During aging, humans and other mammals become increasingly inelastic in their skin and arteries. This inelasticity is largely the result of oxidation (O) of the chemical bond (=N) which holds collagen and elastin fibers rigidly together. This oxidation is a process leading to permanent cross-links between fibers, as depicted at the bottom of this drawing. Cross-linking can be partially reversed with carnosine treatment.

Skin Protection against Photo (Sunlight) Aging
Please feed your skin and eyes with nutrients such as carnosine that will partially reverse collagen cross-linking.

Everyone knows it is important to protect skin and eyes from the sun. The sun's *UVA* radiation ages the skin, the sun's *UVB* radiation burns it, and both cause the skin to wrinkle. UVA becomes the more energetic of the two since it resonates at a lower wavelength and therefore it can more easily penetrate down deep and cause havoc even in the most remote parts of your skin's dermis. Your dermatologist can clearly see this cross linking with a special viewing instrument which allows in-depth viewing and predicting what your skin will look like twenty years in the future.

The sun damages the lens of the eye, and therefore, please shield the eyes with a 100% *UV* (ultraviolet) protection-marked sun glasses. Be preventive and do not buy fashion sunglasses. Also, refrain from buying sunglasses that do not wrap around on the sides or are excessively dark. Very dark glasses open your pupils wider than normal and allow in extra quantities of the sun's UV radiation. Sitting in the shade under an umbrella on a beach or in a boat will not protect your eyes and skin. UV glare from water will reflect and penetrate your eyes and skin.

In conclusion, remember that it is important to protect your skin and eyes from sunlight with proper shading and protective blocking lotions. On the other hand, you need some sunlight since the skin produces essential Vitamin D3, especially during winter months. In addition, please feed your skin and eyes with nutrients such as carnosine that will help to reverse the skin's collagen cross-linking.

Golden keys to longevity #9

- *Use carnosine for preventing cross linking and hardening of the skin and lens of the eyes. Use hyaluronic acid lotion and capsules for optimal moisturization of the skin. Use lithium orotate for skin itching and minor nerve problems. Use strong antioxidants for protecting against photo aging of the skin and natural hyaluronic acid cream for moisturizing.*

Chapter 10
Health Despite Pollution

What to Do?

"We have earthquakes, landslides, industrial pollution, tobacco smoke, smog & acid rain . . . If you die of natural causes, it's considered an accident!" Johnny Carson

Since most scientific reports focus on pollution effects upon children and pregnant women, we lack health-risk data with regard to the adult population. For example, the levels of lead and mercury in our bodies have become a thousand times greater than the levels humans had a mere four hundred years ago. I believe that *any* level of a heavy metal is toxic to us. Scientists and concerned laymen have made only educated guesses as to the effects of pollutants in our environment.

Take cancer. Most human cancers are caused by choices that we make regarding our environment and lifestyle, and not by involuntary exposure to pollutants. We can choose to improve our health and reduce pollution risks by simple means. Tobacco smoke and *smoked meat and fish* have become as great a danger to our health as all other environmental pollutants combined. Each cigarette inhalation means exposure to billions of cancer-causing molecules called *benzopyrines*. It only takes one of these molecules to react in a normal cell and cause irreversible cancer.

Tars, Tobacco, Smoked Foods, and Protectives
"My Prius runs on fruit and pebbles, and my sandals are made of spirulina." Dana Carvey

Tars in tobacco and smoked fish and meat contain polyaromatic (many chemical rings) hydrocarbons or PAHs. In humans, PAHs become cancer causing agents (carcinogens) by a process in our cells called *epoxidation*. Epoxidized PAHs cause 40 to 80% of all human cancers through initiating changes or mutations in our genetic material or DNA. Another unwanted change is the formation of atherosclerotic plaques (*damaged arteries*) from the huge amount of carbon monoxide in cigarette and diesel smoke. Plaques even cause blood clotting, stroke and heart failure.

Tars in cigarette smoke are extremely dangerous. Tobacco and its burnt PAHs have caused the untimely deaths of Ingrid Bergman, Humphrey Bogart, Steve McQueen, Sammy Davis Jr. and John Wayne. Unfortunately, the typical smoker consumes as much tar from low-tar as from high-tar cigarettes since a smoker unconsciously learns to inhale more deeply and puff more frequently in order to get the same amount of tar.

The cancerous effects of tobacco and smoked meat and fish can be somewhat reduced by consuming antioxidant nutrients such as methionine, cysteine, selenium, glutathione, and Vitamins C and E. But I would not bet my life on it. These nutrients remain slightly effective against *nitrate* toxins produced by automobiles, natural gas ovens and heaters, and Viagra®. The latter is a free-radical generator of *nitrous oxides*. At home, antioxidants protect somewhat against nitrates (*nitrosoamines*) in bacon, baloney, sausage, beer and snuff. Beer contains far fewer nitrates than bacon, but we consume much more of it. Interestingly, if you soak ordinary raw, red-colored bacon in warm water for an hour, it will return to its natural silvery-grey color since the nitrosoamines have leached out into the water! I do not find this natural color pleasing to the eye, but I have grown accustomed to it.

A friend asked me how full-time or passive smoking affects the body. I said that after about four minutes large blood vessels begin to stiffen and lose their elasticity. After about a half hour, the membranes of red blood cells began to break down and become sticky. This stickiness results in blood clots which damage arteries and may cause stroke. Finally, after several hours of smoking, heart rhythm becomes more erratic, a phenomenon called *"arrhythmia"*. For example, my good friend, Chester Young died last year because his smoking had given him undiagnosed arrhythmia.

Another friend of mine read the foregoing and asked me what I meant by the adverse consequences of smoked meats and fish. I answered they had become a tasty favorite of many, but they contain some inherent dangers. While attending medical school many years ago, I studied a medical crisis in an Icelandic fishing village during 1948. *In this village, 60% of the population developed stomach cancer from their smoked-fish preserving activities.* Unfortunately, this important study and similar ones have been largely ignored in the US. For similar reasons, Japanese living in Japan have three times the rate of stomach cancer than Japanese immigrants in the US due to high intake of smoked fish sauces and soups. Indeed, in my family my grandfather died from seafood carcinogens since he loved smoked foods, especially oysters. Apparently, the differences remain insignificant between PAHs in your lungs from cigarette smoke and PAHs in your stomach or intestines from eating smoked fish or meat.

Perhaps 90% of all lung cancers are caused by cigarette smoke. Sixty years of scientific data have confirmed the above, and yet ignorance persists.

Chlorinated Water
These substances in the drinking water may even contribute to hardening of the arteries.

Chlorination of the public water supply has become a necessity in preventing common maladies of the Third World such as dysentery and cholera. But perhaps preventing maladies of the *First* World with chlorine should also become a health goal. Perhaps. During 2006, the sewage overflows in New Orleans and Honolulu went untreated due to government inaction. These overflows should have been sprayed with a weak Clorox® solution. Consequently, I sometimes wonder if we do live in a Third World country given the typical unresponsiveness of government during the last 7 years.

Of course, using Clorox® would have violated EPA, OSHA, MENSA, NASA and FDA guidelines, *but in an emergency*, the health of every citizen should be protected with whatever means at hand. As everyone discovered in the aftermath of hurricane Katrina, government remains unresponsive to the average citizen, especially those agencies enmeshed in bureaucratic red tape.

However that may be, both chlorinated water and Clorox® contain the interesting ingredient, *hypochlorite* which easily converts to the extremely strong oxidant or pro-oxidant, *chlorine dioxide*. Chlorine dioxide provides chlorinated water with its cleaning and anti-bacterial properties. But these substances in the drinking water may even contribute to hardening of the arteries previously described. Although never scientifically proven, chlorinated tap water may well contribute to your ill health and aging. Chlorinated water blocks iodine uptake, critical to thyroid function and avoiding cancer.

In my experiments at the Department of Medical Cell Biology in Sweden, *I was first to discover that I could easily deactivate both hypochlorite and chlorine dioxide by using various strong antioxidants. I also determined that doing so can have a positive effect in brain and liver cells.* They can be removed from tap water by simple filtration or deionization devices available at building supply stores. Alternatively, I recommend glass-bottled water such as my Swedish favorite, "*Ramlösa*"; although some bottled waters may have high bacteria counts. Interestingly, both hypochlorite and chlorine dioxide enhance the chemical reactivity of hydrogen peroxide common in hair dye and some processed foods.

Hydrogen Peroxide in the Body
The body protects us against it with the special enzyme, catalase that deactivates it.

When accidentally spilled, a typical 3% hydrogen peroxide solution turns one's skin a sickly white. Hydrogen peroxide remains damaging to healthy cells, but ironically, the body produces it in enormous amounts as a normal byproduct of oxygen metabolism. The body protects us against it with the special enzyme, *catalase* that deactivates it. For this reason, I have often incorporated catalase into several of my anti-aging formulas. For example, *ACF 228 ™* contains catalase useful in destroying peroxides ingested with food.

Catalase will destroy hydrogen peroxide over a wide range of acidity and alkalinity, especially in the highly acidic environment of the stomach. On the other hand, supplemental intake of the enzyme, SOD (*superoxide dismutase*) remains unworkable in the stomach or blood stream where it might do some good. The SOD molecule is enormous in size, and therefore, it cannot penetrate the stomach and intestinal linings. It can only be injected. But in that case, white blood cells treat it as a foreign invader and destroy it. However, physicians in Europe have used external treatment with SOD to treat severe radiation burns.

ACF 228 ™ or "Aging Control Formula 228" is the one and only antiaging nutrient mixture registered with two governmental medical authorities. It was duly examined, approved and registered by both the Swedish and Italian FDAs. This is especially significant since the Swedish FDA has the most difficult registration requirements in Europe, if not the world. www.antiaging-motivate.com

Hypochlorite and Transition Metals
Heavy-metal concentrations in our body fat have become so high that if we could eat our own fat, we would probably die from heavy metal poisoning.

Hypochlorite and its near cousin, chlorine dioxide, have enhanced reactivity with different transition metals such as iron, copper, cobalt, manganese and zinc. For this reason, I do not recommend supplementing these metals in our diet but for two exceptions: lactating women who need extra iron, and men with prostate difficulties who perhaps need extra zinc.

Fortunately, you can minimize heavy metal pollution by consuming sulfur-containing antioxidants such as methionine, cysteine, and glutathione. These sulfur-containing antioxidants *chelate* (absorb and deactivate) heavy metals with their free sulphur groups. These groups easily chemically bind with toxic metals such as arsenic, mercury, and lead. Then the body excretes or stores them.

Interestingly, amino acids, glutathione and similar sulphur-containing medications have helped to reverse autism in the Hawaiian Islands. Scientists suspect that high mercury intake from the environment may have contributed to autism. Glutathione remains an effective chelator of mercury, and certainly high mercury intake may add to other ailments in our modern industrial society.

The body often neutralizes the toxic effects of heavy metals through fat storage, which should concern everyone with a bulging midriff. During the last fifty years, heavy-metal concentrations in our body fat have become so high that if we were to eat our own body fat, we would probably die from heavy metal poisoning! Part of the problem stems from the frequent use of leaded gasoline used in past decades from which *tetraethyl lead* stored itself in our body fat. Fortunately, the government phased out this lead during the early nineties.

The release of heavy metals into the blood stream perhaps accounts for euphoric or depressive effects experienced during dieting or fasting. This occurs when body fat becomes metabolized. Antioxidants or EDTA should rid the body of heavy metals that become sequestered in the fatty walls of our arteries. During acute, heavy metal poisoning, EDTA tablets are prescribed, and I myself often ingest a half gram to cleanse my arteries as an on-going means of prevention.

Further supplementing with potassium iodine will prevent thyroid problems since it competes with *radioactive iodine* from nuclear fallout.

Nuclear Proliferation
Potassium iodine will compete with radioactive iodine from nuclear fallout and prevent problems with one's thyroid.

In the event of another Chernobyl disaster, the radioactive substance, *strontium 90* and other byproducts will appear in the environment. Strontium 90 follows the calcium pathway in our bodies. This means that its presence in our bodies would make our bones brittle, and we may suffer from leukemia. Mexicans use one of the world's best natural protections against strontium 90 and other nuclear byproducts by consuming daily large quantities of calcium hydroxide in their corn-rich diets. Calcium hydroxide in the form of *corn* tortillas is an important natural source of pure calcium in the prevention of osteoporosis, especially if combined with high-dose Vitamin D3. Secondly, this hydroxide is a strong base effective in precipitating and eliminating unwanted strontium 90. Eating a corn-rich Mexican diet provides some protection, but in the aftermath of another Chernobyl, stronger medicines become essential. In such an awful event, protection may be achieved by 10 milligrams daily of *Kryptofix™* and avoidance of all dairy products. Other medicines include *Lewisite*, *penicillamine* and other sulphur-containing antioxidants, but EDTA will work similarly to these drugs. They work by binding or chelating heavy metals in our bodies. As explained previously, radiation generates high doses of free radicals in the body, and these sulphur-containing compounds inhibit most radicals. These should be consumed orally with iodine and iodide tablets such as *Ioderal* from vrp.com.

To my knowledge, no company produces a Chernobyl-type survival kit. Such a kit would also include antibiotics, burn ointment, tranquillizers, pain killers, and vaccines against epidemics.

Another Chernobyl would require a survival kit containing protective UV glasses and suits sealing off our bodies. Definitely no fun. Australians already use heavy protective creams and clothing in response to lack of ozone protection in the southern hemisphere. As suggested earlier, we could obtain some protection by bathing daily in the chelator EDTA which I regularly recharge in my shower's filter. Interestingly, when it comes to radiation, cockroaches are naturally the most resistant species to it since they have thick shells

185

made of *keratin* and naturally retain high levels of antioxidant protection.

Golden Key to Longevity #10

- *Consume a minimum of 250 mg of strong antioxidants with every meal to deactivate many environmental pollutants. If you are a sun worshipper, bathe weekly in a two gram bath of EDTA to chelate out unwanted metals. Eat Mexican corn foods.*

Recommendations:

- Eat fresh, raw or semi-raw fish, and avoid burnt or smoked fish, oysters, meats, and tobacco.
- 250 mg/d l-methionine, l-cysteine, N-acetyl-cysteine, Vitamins C, E, and D, selenium, BHT, and/ or ACF 228.
- Nitrates in all processed meats, e.g. bacon, baloney, sausage, and some types of beer and snuff.
- Clean with Clorox. Drink glass-bottled or filtered water. Chelate with EDTA. Eat Mexican corn tortillas.

Chapter 11
Use It Or Lose It!

A Nitty-Gritty Love, Pain and Exercise Guide

"Cialis: There should be a warning label on it. Otherwise you end up having sex with someone you shouldn't!" Jay Leno

Men – Introduction
"Typically, an older man is still interested in sex, and he jumps at an idea that here's a pill he can take orally that will make him a new man. The trouble is his wife is no longer interested . . . . So her husband is all dressed up with nowhere to go." Dr. Klorfein

Many men over the age of 50 seem disappointed that they do not feel young anymore. They could feel young again and regain the energy of lost youth if mainstream medicine would take aging seriously. The worst symptom of aging is the loss of sexual activity due to both loss of sexual function and appetite. Mainstream medicine should step aside and let physicians specializing in anti-aging medicine help those with aging problems.

Most men advancing in age have some degree of sex-organ

atrophy. During aging, men lose over fifty percent of their Leydig cells in their testes, and these cells produce most of a man's testosterone (T). Indeed, men over 45 may have low *free* T while their *total* T shows normal. And worse, the little free T they do possess gets converted to *estradiol* – a female hormone! Women need some estradiol for normal health, but men should minimize it to avoid *feminization*. Late in life, no true man wants to become *effeminate*. Men can remedy this situation by doing the following:

- First, men advancing in age should be blood tested both for free testosterone and SHBG or sex-hormone binding globulin. Alternatively, they can take an extremely comprehensive *24-hour urine test without prescription* at www.meridianvalleylab.com. I strongly recommend the latter since it directly reveals *free* T values without any approximations or calculations.

- Second, these men should reinstate testosterone back to the normal levels of younger men with bio-identical gels or cream formulated by a *compounding* pharmacy. This type of pharmacy employs specialty pharmacists who custom blend to order gels or creams to the requirements of individual customers. Check your local phone book.

- Third and forth, men should take DIM (*di-indoylmethane*) daily to prevent excess estradiol and feminization. A more long-term approach even employs *aromatase blockers* that lower female hormones. My favorites are the herb *chysin (50mg twice daily in cream or nasal spray)* or the drug *Arimidex™* (0.1 mg twice weekly orally or in cream form.) They have the advantage of preventing two carcinogens that are responsible for breast, uterine, and possibly even prostate cancers. I advise a tiny dose of 0.1 mg 2X weekly since higher doses can cause joint and bone pain.

- Fifth, some sexual atrophy can be reversed by using Viagra™ , or my favorite, Cialis™. However, these drugs only address the symptoms, and thus, I recommend the superior medical practice of addressing the *causes* by using the aforementioned therapies.

- Sixth, for senior men only, I strongly recommend increasing libido with Deprenyl™ at 15 mg per week which has wonderful side benefits such as increased focus and attention.

- Seventh, please men, use only 10 mg daily in the morning of DHEA.
- Eighth and last, my absolute best tip for enhancing erections employs 10 international units (iu) sublingually of the hormone *oxytocin*. For daily maintenance of hormone balance, I recommend 5 iu. Women have used this hormone successfully since 1913, but only recently researchers have discovered positive benefits for men. Oxytocin compliments testosterone by providing men with *rock-hard erections throughout intercourse*. Postcoitually, it also helps men and women to bond emotionally with one another. This is my Dr. Lippman Promise.

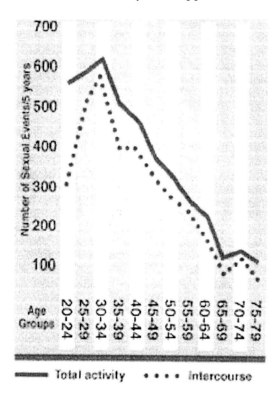

Figure One. Sexual activity of men declines sharply after age 30. (supplied by Ward Dean, MD)

Women – Introduction

Most women switched from the horse-excrement hormones to bio-identicals, especially estriol, and the following year's results demonstrated dramatic drops in breast and ovarian cancers.

"After an hour she began to feel "a fullness. I can't say it was a tingling, but it was some effect of the increased blood flow to the area." 42 year old nurse using Viagra®

Any physician prescribing the aforementioned drugs should question his male patients regarding the age of their sexual partners. If their female partners are older than 45, they likely lack some estrogens accompanied by vaginal dryness, itching and pain. These symptoms are easily remedied by applying to the vagina *estriol* cream or gel available from compounding pharmacies or without prescription outside of the US.

The older women become, the more likely intercourse involves vaginal dryness and even pain. Fortunately, several remedies address this situation:

- Use vaginal creams using only bio-identical estrogens from a compounding pharmacy two to three times weekly. Bio-identical hormones are preferred since other synthetic and horse hormones may increase heart problems and cancer. This is the underlying message of the Women's Health Initiative Report in 2002.
- Women should use my favorite, *Esnatri®,* invented by the famous Harvard grad, Jonathan Wright, M.D. In cream form, it contains bio-identical triple estrogens close to a woman's natural ratios of 80% estriol, 7% estradiol, and 13% estrone. An 80% estriol mixture is employed since this estrogen has definite anti-cancer properties. It helps to eliminate the carcinogens, namely the *4 and 16 alpha hydroxyestrones.* Esnatri is available off-shore and without prescription at www.antiaging-motivate.com. Please note that Esnatri and other estrogen products should be used with cancer blockers such as the previously mentioned Arimidex or chysin.

190

- Women over 45 years old should also use 50 mg daily of DHEA for improvement of sexual response and alleviation of hypertension.
- Women would also benefit from 150-300mg bio-identical progesterone cream, especially if their 24-hour urine tests indicate a deficiency.

Bio-identical hormones are the only practical way to avoid stroke, blood clots, and cancer. For these reasons, drug companies selling other types of artificial hormones have lost many of their customers in recent years. These "other types" I call the space-alien-abortion hormones since they are made from horse excrement or have never before been seen on planet Earth. It is your life and your choice, but I believe that you should avoid intimidating doctors who willingly swallow the advertising pitches of drug reps touting space-alien hormones.

Indeed, some physicians I know deny entry to drug reps in their offices since these docs have switched to a more natural, bio-identical approach. Use some common sense and chose bio-identical hormones. When the Women's Health Initiative report was issued in 2002, most women changed from the *horse-excrement hormones* to bio-identicals, especially natural *estriol* and *progesterone*, and the following year's results *demonstrated dramatic drops in breast and ovarian cancers*. In other words, some forms of cancer are preventable if you find help from a knowledgeable physician. In Sweden, women have a *political right to buy estriol without prescription* at any pharmacy. Swedish women realized that estriol effectively defends against breast and uterine cancers.

Additionally, both sexes should keep sexually active since if we do not use it, we lose it. And this statement especially applies to women who begin using vaginal creams before menopause rather than afterwards.

The Pain-Relieving Miracles of Creatine and DMSO
Simply roll it on a painful muscle group, and within ten minutes, most pain and stiffness will disappear.

If you are over the age of 45, you may have awakened some mornings and found muscle aches and pains. Everyone gets aches and pains as a natural result of aging. Do not worry unless you are experiencing pain from *hormonal imbalances*, particularly those involving the hormones thyroid and cortisol. Other examples are the *statin drugs* used for high cholesterol which have a serious side-effect which causes muscle weakness due to depletion of *coenzyme Q10.*

I have two easy solutions for the everyday aches and pains in your muscles. I take *creatine* 750 mg capsule or powder daily, available at better health food and sports stores. Most muscle pains will disappear after about 45 minutes if taken on an empty stomach. Then, take a half-hour walk to stretch your muscles. This method will truly work since athletes use it routinely. Creatine stokes your energy pump and increases conversion of *ADP* (adenosine diphosphate) to *ATP* (adenosine triphosphate). ATP is the "gasoline" of your muscles, and the more available ATP you have, the more strength and endurance your muscles will have. An ATP shortage may result in muscle aches and pains. I sometimes experience morning aches and pains if I have exercised heavily the previous day. In fact, creatine is so effective *in stoking* the ADP to ATP pump that you only need one-third the normal ADP to produce an *abundance of ATP*. My favorite source of creatine is called Mitoboost I™ from www.vrp.com. Mitoboost #I provides a pleasant morning breakfast drink when mixed with a little fruit juice.

A second product, *DMSO roll-on*, is a great little treatment for highly localized pain in a specific muscle group. Try Googling "DMSO roll-ons". Several companies sell DMSO (dimethyl sulfoxide) in a roll-on applicator through the internet. Simply roll it on a painful muscle group, and within ten minutes, most pain and stiffness will disappear. You will know that DMSO is working and has penetrated the skin when your breath smells a bit like garlic, since it quickly absorbs in the blood stream and becomes excreted partially through the lungs. It can also be used to increase the rate of absorption of the aforementioned hormone creams, but I do not recommend it.

A third remedy applies 30 mg of progesterone cream to sore muscles. Progesterone is anti-inflammatory and a natural method to reduce pain and alleviate inflammation.

Nutrition and Sex
Senior sex life will be enhanced by this simple nutritional trick.

In seniors, hormones and muscles will refuse to work well when a proper diet is lacking. During one's senior years, poor nutrition and lack of vitamins, especially the B vitamins, can precipitate health disasters. During aging, poor nutrition has become a real problem. Many seniors personally known to me eat sugary cereal or "health bars" for breakfast (yuk) instead of a truly healthy breakfast consisting of eggs, fish or baked beans (Bush) on toast and not "sugar bars" and breakfast meats. Many seniors lose mealtime interest since they have lost half their taste buds and smell sensors between age 35 and 70. A lack of proper food interest is murder for one's health, sex life, and longevity. Trust me. My best remedy is to position seniors next to a stove when cooking to allow pleasant aromas from the steaming food to enter their nostrils. This method increases secretion of gastric juices and enzymes and promotes pangs of hunger. My unique method also works with children who are finicky eaters.

During 1977, my oldest son Sebastian refused to eat. I assigned him the job of stirring and turning over frying fish or meat. His nostrils and stomach reacted to the aromatic cooking smells, and after participating for about ten minutes, he was ready to eat with robust appetite. It truly works in people of all ages. Senior sex life will be enhanced by this simple nutritional trick.

Exercise and Sex
"Nature wants us to be horny and spread seed!
When you're 75, you should be thinking about God and not
shagging the lady next door!" Comedian Bill Maher

"Older people are having more sex thanks to Viagra and no risk of
pregnancy. Sexually transmitted diseases are becoming rampant!
My question is: Where are the parents?" Comedian Jay Leno

A top biologist in aging research is Professor Raj Sohal. He experiments with houseflies and finds that highly sexually active flies do shorten their lifespans by about fifty percent. Fortunately, the opposite holds true in humans. We need exercise to keep healthy, and Mother Nature has given us a complex set of free-radical defenses that rid our bodies of toxins acquired while exercising. In fact, exercise remains the only way to keep a healthy heart and digestive system functioning properly. Case in point is my dear friend, Chester, who died last year at age 59. He never did much exercising except an occasional short walk. If one plans to survive long into the 21st century, one needs real exercise and not short strolls to the supermarket.

By real exercise, I mean taking 4 to 6 hour walks whenever possible. At age 63, I do real exercise which means 3 hours of housework or one hour of tree trimming with ladders and power saws. Or perhaps a half hour of vigorous sports activities such as cycling (my favorite). An absolute minimum should be a half hour daily combined with sensible food and antiaging supplements. As my grandparents used to say, real exercise and work are truly worthwhile since a healthy mind can only rest upon a healthy body. Getting enough exercise remains key to healthy aging as long as one avoids the farm-hand portions of most restaurants. This and lack of real exercise will devastate your body.

Thirty minutes of moderate activity every day helps to manage weight and reduce stress, increase energy, boost the immune system, lower blood pressure and cholesterol, and enhance sex life. Secondly, I take a quarter grain of Amour thyroid hormone prophylactically to raise my metabolism to high normal instead of merely normal. This remedy is a vital key to optimal health, energy, and weight control.

194

In the words of comedian George Burns: "Keep a young mind and a healthy body. I have a young mind, and I'm taking a healthy body to dinner tonight."

Enhanced Romance
Arginine intake of 500 mg daily causes increased lustfulness in women, especially if combined with 4 to 7 mg daily of bio-identical testosterone cream.

Sometimes a healthy body and sex life depend upon taking a younger mate. Nature has often programmed us to think and act in this manner despite social pressures to the contrary. In other countries, the taking of a younger mate remains completely natural. For example, in southern India, some communities encourage polygamy in which one woman is married simultaneously to several younger husbands. (And you thought that only happened among certain orthodox Mormons.) Many industrial countries not only permit a younger mate, but encourage it. For example, Parisian women in their sixties sometimes dress themselves in the fashionable clothing of twenty year olds. A strange and wonderful world.

I should mention the case of former French President François Mitterrand. A reporter on his death bed asked him about his young mistress. He replied with a Gaelic shrug of his shoulders: "So what"? Is the world wrong and Americans always right? I think not. Sex and strange relationships are cornerstones of being human.

Happy and healthy people realize the close relationship between exercise, sex, and weight reduction; if you want any one of these three things, you should try to address all three areas. Weight reduction will enhance your self esteem and sex drive. Combine dieting with increased sexual activity, and you will further your goals of a healthy, happy life. The French are right. Some nutrients help increase sexual activity and reduce weight. For women, I advise 250 milligrams twice daily of *arginine* from Twin Labs. Arginine functions by increasing the metabolism of the *Krebs cycle*, especially effective in the outer skin layers. For this reason, arginine may help to eliminate some cellulite since this skin problem often remains unresolved by dieting or exercising. Since arginine increases skin metabolism, taking 500 mg daily causes increased lustfulness in women, especially if combined with 4 to 7 mg daily of bio-identical testosterone cream applied to their labia. This works, ladies. The same may be true of the previously mentioned topical vaginal creams. Hold your horses and do not use those ill-conceived horse-excrement or space-alien remedies. Your sex life is at stake.

Secondly, dysfunctional women should try consuming 12 units sublingually of the hormone *oxytocin* available only at University pharmacy in San Diego. Oxytocin is known as the "bonding hormone" since mono-orgasmic women become multi-orgasmic. Also women without much interest in sex find new horizons of sexual pleasure by employing it.

Besides oxytocin, Viagra™, and Cialis™, men can also benefit by increasing their amount of ejaculate. Try 80 mg of zinc combined with 100 *micrograms* of selenium. This will put lead in your pencil, men. At the other extreme, one should avoid loss of ejaculate AND LIBIDO by refusing *Proscar®* or *finasteride*. Instead, substitute with 30 mg daily of natural progesterone cream rubbed vigorously on the testicles. I also strongly recommend one capsule twice daily of "Prostate Essentials Plus" from www.swansonvitamins.com .

Also, as mentioned previously, both sexes should try a spray-snort of the prescription drug, *Diapid®* (lysine-vasopresin) before intercourse. Lastly, an interesting alternative employs injections of human growth hormone (HGH). HGH rev-starts a cascade of hormones in the body. HGH will up-regulate every hormone by acting on the body's juvenile cells, especially when combined with bio-identical testosterone cream. It even encourages weight loss more blood flow to the pelvic region of the body – a necessity for an active and functional sex life.

I also recommend another well known pharmaceutical named *Deprenyl®*. Deprenyl has aphrodisiac effects by helping to improve sexual function and desire. I advise 3 mg daily, and it may be purchased offshore without prescription at www.antiaging-motivate.com.

Final Thoughts
Some forms of cancer can be prevented by ingesting 0.1 mg twice weekly of Arimidex.

If you have doubts about HGH, oxytocin, testosterone, Viagra and vaginal creams, there is always good old fashioned *coffee*. Interestingly, coffee was a *controlled substance* during the eighteenth century as depicted in the wood cut below. Commonly available today are strong coffee and espresso. They remain excellent euphorics that may enhance your sex life. However, coffee does elevate adrenaline, cortisol (the stress hormone), and cytokines (inflammatory proteins). Therefore, I avoid using it especially in stressed-out patients with adrenal problems. Instead, I encourage patients to switch to green tea powder sweetened with xylitol sugar and a dash of soy milk. The Chinese have used antioxidant-rich green tea for millennia. Chairman Mao swore by the health benefits of green tea, and during his senior years he pleased four mistresses.

Another interesting enhancer for women is *estradiol*. Interestingly, I can identify young women who naturally possess lots of estradiol by the rosiness of their cheeks, the wideness of their hips, and the perky firmness of their breasts. Nature intended these estradiol benefits for libido, fertility, and the propagation of the specie. In aging women, estradiol reinstatement likewise increases libido, especially when combined with testosterone and applied daily to labia. As a side benefit in aging women, estradiol applied to facial wrinkles encourages their reduction. This one tip alone will save some women from needless trips to a plastic surgeon. However, estradiol use remains a double-edged sword since it must be balanced diligently with 30 mg or more daily of natural progesterone cream to avoid *hyperplasia* (cell growth) of ovarian, breast, as well as prostate tissues.

Last but not least is affection. Everyone needs affection and human physical contact, and here is where the natural bonding hormone oxytocin plays a vital role for enhanced health, libido, and sexual happiness.

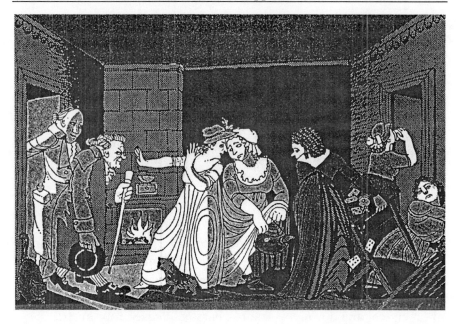

Figure Two. Coffee was illegal in Sweden from 1756 to 1822, and the police often made search and seizure raids for this highly stimulating, illicit drug. This was another "war on drugs" event as later experienced in twentieth century America.

Golden Key to Longevity # 11

- *Exercise religiously at least a half-hour daily and during aging, use bio-identical <u>natural</u> hormone replacement therapy, especially testosterone in men and estradiol plus progesterone in women, and oxytocin for both.*

Recommendations

- **Men:** Use one to two capsules daily *Prostate Essentials* and 75 mg/d *DIM*. Hormone replacement therapy including 30-100 mg/d bio-identical testosterone combined with 30 mg/d progesterone.

- **Women:** bio-identical hormones. If indicated, vaginal creams such as *Esnatri®* bio-identical triple estrogens and *progesterone*. Always combine with 0.1 mg 2X weekly of Arimidex. Also, 250 mg daily arginine. 50 mg/d *DHEA*. For men: bio-identical testosterone, 80 mg zinc, 100 mcg selenium, and 10 mg/d DHEA. For both men and women: testosterone plus HGH therapy if deficient.

Chapter 12
Beat Indigestion and Inflammation

Honest Help Has Arrived!

"This book is written on self absorbent paper with a built in medic alert." Jay Leno

My patient, Jenny C, 38, interviewed with me and explained in detail her medical history. I had known her for ten years, and had always found her very sociable, lively, and happy. Then, at age 32, her health care provider diagnosed her with hypertension and inflamed bowels. He wrote a prescription for a well-known anti-hypertension drug and recommended changes in diet. She followed the advice only sporadically, and three years later she married a Californian who insisted on eating the typical North American diet rich in inflammatory foods, especially junk burgers, greasy fries, canned tuna, and thick sirloin steaks. This diet was inflammatory because of the loads of *histamine* producing foods.

Jenny's symptoms worsened despite medication. Once, she became angry with me when I suggested that the canned tuna she ate contained high mercury. Canned tuna is one reason why residents of Honolulu have three times the national average of mercury in their bloodstreams. Mercury causes nerve damage and a host of other minor illnesses that people often take for granted as part of growing old. A great pity.

Another time she became distressed when I gently chided her for buying undercooked turkey still pink on the inside. Poultry must be cooked thoroughly at 160 degrees Fahrenheit, until the interior is no longer pink if one wishes to avoid *trichinosis* and bacteria. Jenny had a tendency towards irritation when people offered her opinions that opposed her own.

Then crisis struck. At age 36, she gave birth to a baby girl, and a year later she had her first heart attack. Friends and I tried everything possible to induce her to alter her diet, but to little avail. She was caught in the web of the unhealthy North American diet and flatly refused to change. Finally I asked her point blank who would care for her child if she suddenly died. She remained unconcerned since she had a large life insurance policy that would provide for the child. I replied that her child would definitely want her future help and guidance instead of money. As usual, she became obstinate and in complete conflict with my *Picasso Principal*. A great shame.

I know that I could help her with simple dietary measures as described previously, especially 50,000 units of Vitamin D3 weekly for her hypertension. Perhaps she will change her mind someday and heed my advice before the inevitable occurs. Unfortunately, she is headed for several heart attacks despite her young age.

Inflammation and Digestion
Many people become partially disabled with bad digestion

If you are a person over forty and do not already suffer from an irritable bowel, the odds become fifty-fifty that you will suffer from this affliction by age sixty. By age sixty-five, most Americans have some discomfort with their digestion. The Mayo Clinic and John Hopkins discovered the reason in thousands of seniors, namely low stomach acid called HCl or hydrochloric acid. Low HCl and high cortisol (the stress hormone) causes the gut to become inflamed, and the passage of food from start to finish becomes more difficult and sometimes painful. Absorption of essential nutrients becomes impaired. Many people become partially disabled with bad digestion and some experience the added embarrassment of either constipation or diarrhea. This means a quick trip home after an otherwise delightful meal at a nice restaurant. Gulping down anti-acids may provide temporary relief, but this remedy does not address the underlying causes, especially my discovery of high cortisol in stomach tissues.

The New York Times reported recently that over 45 million Americans spend over $12 billion annually on their digestion problems. Frequently, an inflamed stomach can lead to ulcers, leaky gut, and even surgery. This type of inflammation may even spread to other areas of the body dependent upon the immune system. Year after year, this type of low-level inflammation affects the health of our entire body.

This chapter details a long term treatment for *IBS* (irritable bowel syndrome) where sufferers can obtain at least 80% relief. I advise starting with short-term treatments while you begin adapting to long-term lifestyle changes. You decide.

Background
The discovery of these nutrients promises help for many sufferers over the age of forty.

Researchers have discovered new natural nutrients that help balance key inflammatory components present in the normal digestive tract. The health of the immune system influences the health of the gut with the help of balanced key antioxidants and enzymes. The discovery of these nutrients promises help for many sufferers over the age of forty at risk for developing unhealthy gastro-intestinal (GI) tracts. Among GI tract sufferers who use these nutrients, scientific evidence indicates a positive effect for the entire gut.

The Gut: The Body's Hidden Organ
The first sign is stomach pain and bloating from bacterial overgrowth.

Over 100 trillion bacteria weighing more than three pounds inhabit a normal intestine. This is truly the largest organ in the body and essential for good health since it aids in vitamin and fatty-acid production, food digestion, fat metabolism, and sugar and starch fermentation. We exist in a symbiotic relationship with these trillions of bacteria, and only through steady absorption of nutrients will we maintain good health. We depend upon a good flora of bacteria. Interestingly, if NASA sent space explorers to the nearest star, *Alpha Centauri* at seven light-years away, those astronauts would need to culture intestinal bacteria in their spacecraft's lab in case their own gut cultures became damaged. Lacking these critical bacteria the astronauts, like any human, might very well die.

The gut's *mucosa,* or surface, absorbs nutrients while acting as a barrier to toxins and macromolecules. Absorption can be altered by infections, stress, toxins, poor diet, and inflammation. These factors increase gut permeability which leads to a dysfunction called "*leaky gut*". In an evil-circle, gut inflammation increases *antigen* (inflammatory factors) penetration to the immune system which in turn leads to more inflammation.

Irritable bowel syndrome (IBS) causes illness and imbalance within our digestive tracts. IBS is often caused by bile insufficiency, low stomach acid, poor mastication, and atrophy of intestinal *villi.* Low stomach acid is particularly significant since 78% of IBS sufferers tested positive for small bowl overgrowth of bacteria. This overgrowth problem causes excessive production of methane and hydrogen gases which patients can remedy by taking one or two doses of the antibiotic *Diflucan®* or the natural remedy *KandidaPlex* by www.vrp.com. Also, one should stop eating all milk products and bread since they may contain yeast.

Researchers report that millions of people live with intestinal problems but they remain unaware of it. The first sign is stomach pain and bloating from bacterial overgrowth. Then it progresses to diarrhea, constipation, or both. Because these symptoms are vague, many remain ignored or go undetected until the disease advances beyond the easy treatment stage.

Four Types of Irritable Bowel Disorders
Yet some of the side effects of prescription drugs are almost as bad as the irritable bowel problem itself.

The four most common intestinal problems are infection, bloating, constipation and diarrhea. Infection often starts in the mouth with the bacteria *S. mutans* or in the stomach with *H. pylori*. These infectious bacteria may travel to other areas of the body, especially the intestine and heart muscle.

When they travel to the intestine, bloating and pain often result. After the age of forty, our immune systems become more dysfunctional. At this age, the gut lacks defenses against bad bacteria, and consequently, the entire digestive tract becomes inflamed. The body tries to compensate by producing extra mucus that partially protects the gastrointestinal walls from infection and inflammation. As a result, critical nutrients, especially Vitamin B12 absorb poorly, and without this vitamin we may fall into the group of 45% of Americans who get Alzheimer's at age 80. Other important nutrients such as magnesium and folate acid are especially lacking in vegetarians. All of this triggers an evil circle that ultimately yields poor health, loss of energy, and a compromised immune system.

Surgery can cause further complications, namely future inflammations since the underlying problems remain unsolved. It makes no medical sense to operate on diseased tissue. Even the newest prescription drugs have limited success in permanently reducing underlying problems of inflammation. Indeed, some prescription drug side effects seem to induce irritable bowel problems itself.

The search for digestive relief is frustrating since no single cause and no effective cure exists, and some doctors become dismissive of their patients' complaints. Other more enlightened doctors treat irritable bowels by replacing deficient nutrients with *bio-identical progesterone* 150 mg daily. Progesterone (not Provera) is an extremely effective and natural anti-inflammatory treatment for bowels as well as other inflamed areas of the body.

Bowels Need More Nutrients than Any Other Organ
The majority of Americans eat food overcooked, processed, or missing essential enzymes.

Many scientists have confirmed that when sufficient enzymes, antioxidants, and acid are present, bad bacteria such as *H. pylori* and *S. mutans* are prevented from doing much damage. Bowel disorders remain much more common in developed countries such as the United States than in third world countries. Several factors explain this unusual fact. Primarily, the majority of American meals are overcooked, processed, or missing essential enzymes. As mentioned previously, a sugary soda or "health bar" for breakfast prevents a healthy start of the day. I strongly recommend lightly grilled eggs or fish. Heavy cooking of food destroys a good portion of the most important nutrients used by the stomach and bowels: enzymes, proteins, fish oils, enzymes, and antioxidants.

Dr. Earl Mindel, Ph.D., R.Ph, and author of the *"Vitamin Bible"* says that most of the enzymes in food are lost in processing, or never exist in substantial amounts due to nutrient-poor soil. The world famous founder of the free-radical theory of aging, Dr. Denham Harman, M.D., Ph.D., professor emeritus at the University Of Nebraska School Of Medicine, told me that some 90% of the population consumes diets deficient in enzymes and antioxidants.

Our stomach and bowels use ten times more of these nutrients than any other organ in the body. As we age, our stomach and bowels lack enzymes, antioxidants, and acid critical to good digestion and health. Many scientists have confirmed that sufficient enzymes, antioxidants, and acid can prevent bad bacteria *H. pylori* and *S. mutans* from doing damage. Furthermore, *H. pylori* infection establishes itself as *major causes a great many gastric ulcers, (1) and up to 89% of all duodenal ulcers. (2)*

Dr. Henry C. Lin of the University of Southern California has found that bad bacteria which normally reside only in the large intestine move into the small intestine where they interfere with digestion. Since the body and its immune system cannot control *H. pylori*, it must be eliminated by other means or this terrible infectious agent will last a lifetime.

Nutrient Eliminates Stomach Inflammation
This ancient treatment eliminated 99% of all H. pylori as evidenced by research.

The ancient Greeks practiced an effective solution for eliminating *H. pylori* from the inhabitants of an island in the Mediterranean. On this island more than two thousand four hundred years ago, Greek doctors such as Hippocrates administered to their patients the sap of the evergreen tree, *Pistacia lentiscus*. This ancient treatment eliminated 99% of all H. pylori as evidenced by later research in modern times (3,4,5,6). Today, we call this tree sap *"Mastic"* and it effectively eliminates *H. pylori* and works in a very *cytoprotective,* or cell protective, manner with respect to the gastric mucosa of the stomach. This cell protection shields against stomach damage caused by prescription drugs and pollutants in the environment.

In total, four prominent research teams published studies confirming Mastic's healing properties for the stomach and intestinal tract. Fortunately, Mastic can be taken orally as a nutritional supplement without prescription. Some doctors call it the "stomach vitamin".

Mastic alone needs the help of another nutrient, *quercetin.* Quercetin works as a powerful inhibitor of *histamine*. Histamine releases from *basophil* and *mast* cells when they encounter allergens. As mentioned previously, bad bacteria or allergy-causing food causes allergens, especially histamine. The addition of quercetin to your diet during the early stages of histamine release results in stopping histamine release (7). Interestingly, many medicinal plants owe much of their activity to their high quercetin content.

The Scientific Explanation of Inflammation
Chronic or "silent" inflammation intimately involves itself in the development of insulin resistance, diabetes, cancer, heart disease, obesity, and Alzheimer's.

Scientists define inflammation as the protective response of body tissues to irritation or injury. Inflammation may become acute or chronic, indicated by signs of swelling, heat, redness, and pain. Scientists often find these symptoms together with loss of tissue function.

For some Americans, inflammation has taken on a life of its own. Inflammation has become self-perpetuating, and a vicious cycle of *chronic* inflammation develops. Chronic or "silent" inflammation intimately involves itself with the development of insulin resistance, diabetes, cancer, heart disease, obesity, and Alzheimer's and other dementias. Consuming daily large quantities of marine omega-3 oils will help to remedy this silent inflammation.

Dominance in our diet of *marine omega-3 oils* over vegetable oils such as corn oils (omega-3s and omega-6s) means that our inflammatory response enzymes, *lipoxygenase (LOX)*, and *cyclo-oxygenase (COX)*, get shut down. Thus, the bad and good oils compete for attention with LOX and COX, and when the good oils dominate, inflammation is reduced. When the bad oils dominate, inflammation increases, and a host of other symptoms arise. Inflammation increases when LOX and COX convert vegetable, dairy product, and red-meat oils into *"eicosanoid oils."*

As deadly oils, these aggressive poisons activate cascades of inflammation. Scientists measure inflammation by two routine clinical tests: *C-reactive protein* (CRP) and *interleukin-6*. A C-reactive protein level lower than 0.5 mg/l is good, but a level of 2 or 3 mg/l remains bad it causes inflammation throughout the body. I keep my own CRP at about 3. An interleukin-6 level below 0.93 pg/ml is good, but a level of 1.50 pg/ml or higher is bad.

No wonder people suffer from a wide variety of swellings, allergies, redness, gastritis, and nauseam. Avoid the poisonous eicosanoid oils by inhibiting LOX and COX enzymes with a diet low in the bad oils and dominant in fish and fish oil.

It works.

The Intestinal Tract Needs Several Nutrients
The ancient Greeks and many other ancient cultures have found many amazing new cures centuries ago.

To insure the health of your intestinal tract, you should provide it with several nutrients: most multiple vitamins, *bromelain, quercetin, deglycyrrhizinated licorice, creosote, Metamucil, dried prunes, Mastic,* and stomach acids such as HCl or my absolute favorite, citric acid in the form of grapefruit juice. These exotic nutrients usefully keep the intestinal tract healthy and have been shown to reduce inflammation in numerous research studies. For example, Vitamin C is a natural *antihistamine* which prevents histamine release and detoxifies histamine already in the body. Large doses of Vitamin C lowers blood histamine levels up to 38% in healthy adults (8).

Doctors G. Kelly and S. Tausig (9, 10) discovered that the proteolytic enzyme, *bromelain* readily absorbs in the bloodstream, and through its action on *fibrin* and *fibrinogen* (clotting factors), bromelain stimulates the production and release of anti-inflammatory *prostaglandin* (Pgs) proteins while simultaneously reducing the production and release of pro-inflammatory Pgs. Furthermore, both bromelain and quercetin work together synergistically in suppressing inflammation caused by food allergens and other sources.

The ancient Greeks and many other old cultures found amazing cures centuries ago. Recently, instead of ignoring them, thousands of prominent scientists have begun searching for every scrap of information about these old medicine-men's secrets. Interestingly, one of the paramount concerns about destroying the tropical rain forests is that some species of plant will disappear that may hold answers to AIDS, cancer, or other diseases.

Dr. F. Pearce and Dr. E. Middleton head up two prominent research groups seeking answers to modern problems. In their laboratories, they found one such answer for digestive disorders. They published their studies in several important medical journals stating that even low levels of quercetin of 10 mg effectively inhibit histamine release. Dr. Pearce and colleagues also explained that "quercetin possesses a broader spectrum of activity than Chromolyn™ (an anti-allergy prescription drug)." (11) Furthermore, Dr. Middleton and associates report that ". . . addition of quercetin during early stages of an ongoing histamine release reaction results in an abrupt cessation of further histamine release." (12)

In other countries, quercetin, bromelain and related *flavonoids* have been used effectively to reduce risk of coronary heart disease. In fact, Dr. Hertog's study of 805 men ages 65 to 84 showed reduced relative risk of coronary heart disease to a 42% level during a five year period by ingesting flavonoids such as quercetin (13).

Dr. D. Stoskes and his colleagues used quercetin in a clinical, double-blind, placebo controlled study. They found that quercetin, in conjunction with bromelain, helped patients with severe and chronic prostatitis (14). Last but not least, quercetin may help to alleviate some forms of cancer. Three independent research teams found that the bioflavonoid quercetin may help to reduce squamous cell carcinoma of the head and neck (15), may inhibit induced mammary cancer (16), and may enhance the anti-cancer effects of several anti-cancer prescription drugs (17).

It is unfortunate that with the availability of these incredible preventatives, most Americans remain unaware of their digestive problems until they become very uncomfortable. Women sufferers seem especially vulnerable to digestive disorders, but they visit doctors more readily than men. Men should heed the same sensitivity since the earlier physicians recognize digestive disorders, the easier the treatment. I advise solving digestive problems by ingesting *Metamucil*, dried prunes, and *Digestif™,* HCl, and pepsin. A viable alternative to HCl is ordinary grapefruit juice, but it definitely should be avoided when consuming prescription drugs. Digestif is available at www.antiaging-motivate.com. Alternatively, in the case of bloating and inflammation, I can also recommend *Advanced Inflammation Control™* or *Cease Fire™* from vrp.com. I am hoping that one day Jenny C. will used these remedies combined with the diet recommendations.

Digestive problems should be of paramount concern to all Baby Boomers who plan to live long and healthy lives well into the 21st century.

Golden keys to longevity # 12

- *For arterial and intestinal health, avoid inflammatory diets, especially for those middle aged and older. From time to time consume Mastic, quercetin, bromelain, Metamucil, licorice, grapefruit juice, and dried prunes for optimal intestinal health.*

Recommended

- Consume fiber with most meals such as Metamucil or Citrucel, 6 g./d.
- Avoid deep fried or greasy food.
- Avoid all processed foods such as cheese, fast food, sugary "health bars."
- Consume fresh, raw foods; oatmeal occasionally, and 4 dried prunes.
- Consume probiotics such as *acidophilus, chlorella, bifida, creosote bush.*
- Use histamine inhibitors such as Vitamin C, *quercetin, bromelain, Mastic,* deglycyrrhizinated licorice (one week only, then rest a week.)
- Try for a general lowering of food allergies by avoiding allergy-causing foods.
- Try for a general lowering of your body's level of inflammation by consuming 6 caps daily of *Oral ChelatoRx* which contains essential minerals, EDTA, chlorella, garlic, malic acid, *gugulipid,* and *serrapeptase.*
- For those over 50, the enzyme pepsin should be combined with extra stomach acids in the form of Vitamin C, HCl, and grapefruit juice in order to maintain stomach acidity (pH) at 4.5 or lower.

Section 3

Personal Finance, Pop Food Culture, & Health Promises Of The New Millenium

Chapter 13
Can You Afford To Live Forever?

Your Health & Long Life Depend upon Your Planning

"If a man empties his purse into his head, no man can take it away from him. An investment in knowledge always pays the best interest." Benjamin Franklin

"As you grow older, the best advice is to be risk adverse!" popular analyst Jim Cramer

I f you live by most of the principles outlined in this book, you are already making a wise financial choice since many of the most expensive and common procedures come as a result of diseases associated with poor lifestyle choices. Also, you do not need to have an unusual or exotic disease in your old age to have financial concerns with respect to health care. Indeed, most health care costs are spent in the last two years of life. These everyday facts of aging and health care cannot be stressed enough.

Medical Emergencies
Most people remain unprepared for medical emergencies despite seemingly complete health insurance plans.

I recently had a pleasant chat with several friends at the Elks Club Lodge overlooking the beautiful beach at Waikiki, Hawaii. Private health care insurance plans were on my mind, and I asked my assembled friends their opinions. Several answered that they had the "premium executive" health care insurance plan which cost about $400 monthly for singles and up to $1,000 for families. Then I asked them if they had read about the plan's benefits.

"I'm covered," they all said.

"I meant the surgery and drug benefits, the maximum benefits and exceptions?" I replied.

"I'm fully covered to $100,000 for drugs alone." they all said in chorus.

"What about the new *biotech* drugs which have become so awfully expensive?" I asked.

"For example, did you know that *Erbitux®* for colorectal cancer initially cost $250,000 for a six month course of treatment? Or Avastin® for lung cancer initially costing $200,000", I questioned.

"Really?" they said, taken aback.

"In fact," I continued, "If your back needs a new, FDA-approved spinal disc from France called a '*Clarité*,' the total fees will exceed $70,000 of which medical insurance covers only about half. Do you have the other $35,000 which insurance does not cover?" I questioned.

Sometimes they said "no," and sometimes "yes," depending on their lifetime habits of spending and saving --- especially saving. The purpose of all my questions and answers was to bring to light the probability that most people remain unprepared for medical emergencies *despite seemingly complete health insurance plans.* They kid themselves into thinking that their HMOs or Medicare supplemental insurance will always pick up the tab. The realities of health care insurance are very different than one may think.

An Investment in Personal Health and Longevity
"There's a growing body of knowledge by hard-nosed economists of all ideological persuasions – University of Chicago, Yale, Harvard, the Rand Corporation – that as societies become more long-living and healthier, that actually creates greater wealth." W. Butler, NIA

What can an American do? Saving more money and investing it correctly remains one solution. A second involves investing in one's personal health with exercise, dieting and the nutrients outlined in this book. Our bodies are our temples, so we should treat them with the same care and reverence as we treat our most holy and revered buildings. Also, we should invest our wisdom and money in our bodies if we plan to live long into the 21st century. We cannot depend on Medicare and private insurance companies for non-medical costs that help to prevent aging and expand longevity.

Furthermore, I remain amazed by people who own several Lexus cars and millions of dollars in real estate but argue with their physicians over a ten-dollar medical insurance copay. Health and longevity costs money, just like these other luxuries. And *if we do not step up to the plate and pay dearly for our health and longevity, then we will be stuck with the marginal solutions that many insurers provide.*

But what can we do about our financial health in coming years? Surely our financial health has become as uncertain as wars, rising gasoline prices, falling real estate and stock prices? Uncertain, yes, but I propose some steps and financial plans to insure a more secure and healthy future:

- **Real Estate.** Real estate always seems to increase in value, decade after decade, despite recessions, wars and inflation. We ought to own our own home free and clear, and if we need money down the road, we can always draw cash from the equity of our own home through a reverse mortgage when we are 62 or older.

- **Reverse Mortgage.** Why would you need a reverse mortgage? Medical emergencies, travel, investment, yes, all of these require money in one's senior years. We especially need to provide for

217

medical emergencies since before the personal bankruptcy laws were changed, *half of all personal bankruptcies left medical bills unpaid.*

- **Credit cards.** What should one do about medical bills if one is without a home that can be reverse-mortgaged? Before you retire and while still working, build yourself a collection of *cash* credit cards. By cash credit cards, I mean Visa, MasterCard, and American Express, and not department store or gas cards. Then only use your cash cards for an occasional purchase to keep them active. If the temptations of one's credit cards become too great, please store them in a safety deposit box -- out of harm's way, so to speak. You may need these cards if you have a serious medical emergency during your senior years.

  Down the road, it is better to max out some of your cards than die through want of funding.

- **Diversification.** With all your investments and money at hand, try to diversify as much as possible. Diversification remains the only free lunch you will ever receive since it spreads risk over a wide variety of different investments. For example, if you own stocks, try to diversify into at least five different industries such as tobacco, technology, energy, commodities, and basic goods and services. Pick stocks that pay well in dividends and wait to buy them when they become out of favor. Regular as clockwork, the stock market sells off *temporarily* at least 10 to 20% twice yearly and even more during recessions such as in the year 2008. This sell-off provides an excellent sign post for investing your hard-earned dollars.

- **A safe investment method.** If you are serious about living long into the 21st century in good health, both medically and financially, I would advise Suzie Orman's method. Suzie Orman started life with two empty hands and a smart head on her shoulders. Currently, her portfolio is valued at $55 million positioned in municipal bonds (munis). Munis typically pay 5 to 8 percent annually and remain free from federal and state taxes. Suzie Orman has the ultimate financial approach to living long into the 21st century.

- **Life insurance.** As we grow older, many of us stop paying our life insurance policies, since the premium is a burden, and our heirs remain without any pressing need for inherited wealth. However, the situation is changing. Elderly people have discovered a new method that insures better financial security for themselves and their love ones. *They need only to cash in on their life insurance policies by selling them to investors.*

  For example, an 80-year old may request investor A to pay a one-year premium of $400,000 on a life insurance policy of six million. If the 80-year old dies within that one year, his heirs and investor A will split the proceeds. For the second and subsequent years, the 80-year old might sell his policy benefits to investor B. In exchange for the full proceeds of the six million, investor B promises to continue paying the $400,000 premium every year. *Also, investor B will pay to the 80-year old 2 million dollars up front.* This wonderful relationship allows the 80-year old immediate benefits — and in today's economy, many elderly have unpaid medical bills, etcetera, which can now be satisfied by this windfall.

- **Negotiate large medical bills.** Some medical procedures can be negotiated for as much as a 74% discount! Believe it. Such remains the case for a cornea transplant at Wills Eye Hospital in Philadelphia which charged $15,000 and that bill was later reduced to $3,900 by an excellent internet company's negotiating. See www.MedicalControl.com. Other medical procedures can typically be lowered by a standard 20%. Recent blood work that I ordered in Honolulu was reduced by 30% merely by asking for their "cash" payment discount. I favor it.

- **A more adventurous approach to life.** What is life without some adventure to it?

  For the more sophisticated investor with long-term holdings of definite blue chip stocks, I would advise finding a stock broker experienced in *writing covered calls*. If your broker were to write covered calls, that is to say, out-of-the-money covered calls against your blue chip stocks, you should realize an extra 15 to 25% income annually. Over eighty percent of all calls expire worthless. This means that your written calls will mostly expire worthless and you pocket the option premiums. For further details, talk to your broker.

If you follow this advice, the worst would be what happened in the case of the extreme bull stock movements during the falls of 2006, 2007, and subsequent 2008 recession. You would forego advancing stock price rises in exchange for some truly fat option premiums. In other words, I prefer the strategy of fat premiums to occasional bonanzas in upward moving stocks. To each his own. Only really savvy brokers know how to implement this covered-call strategy effectively. Choose one and live comfortably long into the 21st century.

In the preceding chapters, I have always advised that one should seek the help of physicians knowledgeable in anti-aging medicine. In the case of one's financial freedom and security, I also advise finding a truly qualified and even certified investment advisor. Some of the best in the country are at Credit Suisse and *Goldman Sachs*. The latter, popularly called "Golden Slacks" remains my favorite.

Golden keys to financial longevity #13

- *Find yourself a knowledgeable investment advisor as well as a knowledgeable anti-aging physician and live long and prosper according to the above strategies. If we do not step up to the plate and pay dearly for our health and longevity, then we will be stuck with the marginal solutions that many health insurers provide.*

Recommendations

- Plan carefully for living long into the 21st century with the help of a professional financial advisor and knowledgeable anti-aging physician.

- Do not assume that your health insurance covers you for all medical problems.
- Own your own home. Reverse mortgage it when necessary. Keep most of your credit cards locked up in a safety deposit box for rainy days.
- Diversify your investments.
- Buy some tax-free muni bonds.

Chapter 14
It's Not Over Until It's Over

A Promise of Healthy Living Long into the 21st Century

"Twenty years from now you will be more disappointed by the things that you didn't do than by the ones you did do. So throw off the bowlines. Sail away from the safe harbors. Catch the trade winds in your sails. Explore. Dream. Discover." Mark Twain

THE FOUR HORSEMEN OF HEALTH

I ride my own carousel of longevity. I invite you to join me, but you will need to choose at least four horses, namely natural bio-identical testosterone, progesterone, oxytocin, and thyroid hormones. These four have nothing to do with horse urine and everything to do with providing your body and its cells with the ultimate in good health. *Without them*, everyone over 50 will suffer many of the indignities of aging long before one's final days on Earth. For example, without adequate testosterone, stiff arteries make one twenty years older. Without adequate thyroid hormone, the risk of dying increases 43% after middle age. Without adequate progesterone sleep suffers and breasts, ovaries, and prostates acquire *hyperplasia* (cell proliferation). Without adequate oxytocin, our sex lives and ability to bond with others suffer.

In addition to these vital four horses, some people will need other hormones for extended or *even normal lifespan*. For example, if your adrenal glands are weak, you may need extra *hydrocortisone*. Secondly in the case of women, they may need extra *estradiol* hormone to retain their femininity (firm breasts) and progesterone to balance it (prevent breast swelling). Thirdly, both men and women with low testosterone and thyroid hormones will experience cardiovascular damage -- forget the hype about cholesterol. Remember that half of all heart attack victims did not have high cholesterol! Fourthly, as a result of a lifetime of free radicals striking the lens of the eyes and causing cross linking (glycation), people should repair the cataract damage by using *N-acetyl carnosine* eye drops and not laser surgery. Fifthly, many will avoid some cancers by using hormone blockers such as *DIM, chrysin,* or very low-dose *Arimidex®*. Sixth, men can simultaneously block both balding and enlarged prostate glands with natural remedies such as progesterone, saw palmetto, etc.

A Hormone Deficiency Case Study
Her appearance betrayed a biological age at least 15 years older than her chronological age.

One day in Stockholm, Sweden I had a friendly conversation with a husband and wife who had health problems. The wife suffered from signs of menopause, but her husband remained contented since he refused to believe in the notion of menopause. Then the wife said that men also get *menopause*. The husband denied it. I intervened and confirmed that men also get a form of menopause, called *andropause*. Andropause is deadly for men since they acquire bulging stomachs and prostates, often balding heads, and cardiovascular disease.

Nearby an acquaintance, Sara H. overheard our heated discussion. Sara sat down next to me and spoke softly in a conspiratorial tone. She had recently celebrated her 36th birthday with her girlfriends of a similar age, and she realized that she did not feel or look as healthy as they did. She whispered that she lacked energy, and was exhausted after an ordinary eight-hour workday. Her situation has become all too common in today's fast-paced modern world. Employing my kindly physician manner, I asked her a few personal questions while examining her hair, eyes, neck and hands. In spite of her 36 years, her appearance betrayed a biological age at least 15 years older than her chronological age. Her hair was dry, brittle and prematurely grey. Her eyes were slightly inflamed and had large black circles beneath them. This indicated pigmentation accented by a line pointing down her cheek in a 4:30 pm direction. I asked her if she also had pigmentation on her elbows. She was surprised that I guessed this simple fact without examining her elbows. Then she became amazed when I asked her if she had a semi-circle of pigment on her shoulder just above her armpit. "Yes," she exclaimed, and she blurted out that I must be some kind of wizard.

"No," I replied, I had only confirmed some classic symptoms of *Addison's* disease. Addison's results in premature aging and death to those who ignore it. I told her that I could help her if she made an appointment for blood work to further confirm my diagnoses. I became confident that she suffered from low cortisol due to weak adrenal glands. Weak adrenals caused her *melanocyte* cells in her skin to produce excess pigmentation in key areas of her body. Indeed, she may have other deficiencies as indicated by her dry, prematurely graying hair. Without hormone replacement therapy, she would rapidly age and die. I could easily solve her immediate problem by administering hydrocortisone tablets 20 mg three times daily. Sara thanked me, and promised to contract me. I was happy to have helped her and others with similar aging problems.

Proper Diet and Supplements
Without these nutritional essentials, your hormones will be short-changed and your life shortened.

Secondly, people need to *support their body's vital hormones* by consuming healthy nourishing food combined with a daily multiple vitamin tablet. **Hormones do not work properly if not supported by healthy nourishing food**, especially fresh fish, eggs, and vegetables.

sugary sodas and so-called "health bars" and increase your of raw fish proteins, oils, iodine, and some fruit. Also, avoid alcohol, caffeine, processed foods, and all forms of sugar. Without these nutritional essentials, your hormones will be short-changed and your life shortened. Hormones will remain dysfunctional and so will your body. Please recall that hormones are the *rate-limiting step* that deficiencies prevent us from living to at least our nineties. Also, remember that if you live in North America, you may well choose to fill your brain with a lifetime of junk burgers, but *only fresh semi-raw fish* allows for a highly functioning brain and body long into your senior years. Indeed, positive diet changes usually correct many hormone problems within 24 hours.

Besides my Caveman, semi-raw diet, you will need daily supplements that *prevent ongoing free-radical damages* to your body. The most important is my **one pill/one meal regimen of truly strong and efficient free-radical scavengers**. Also, you will need other critical *damage-preventing supplements*, especially high dose Vitamin D3 and coenzyme Q10. CoQ10 sustains mitochondrial health in all of your cells, especially the critical non-reproducing cells of the heart, brain, and central nervous system. Vitamin D3 regulates blood pressure by preventing arterial plaques. Indeed, if you must choose between CoQ10 and a multiple vitamin tablet, choose the CoQ10. It is that important.

Thirdly, if over 40, you will need to reverse the body's existing damage with such 21st century longevity aids as *HGH* injections, chelation, *magnesium supplements, mineral and vitamin supports, especially* _methyl_ *folic acid, melatonin, anti-glycators, amino guanidine, resveratrol*, and *N-acetyl carnosine*. For example, HGH therapy is known to repair sagging skin on the buttocks and lower half of the face – all without plastic surgery.

Peripheral Artery Damage
Regular measurement allows accurate assessment and enhancement of your hormones.

In addition to high dose Vitamin D3, everyone with damaged or clogged arteries, especially *peripheral arteries*, should use dietary chelators such as *EDTA* and that brain-cleaning enhancer, *DMSA*. These two wunderkinds cleanse the arteries of heavy metals and some unwanted fats. Also, a cup daily of pomegranate juice may further enhance arteries according to my own experiences and those of Dr. F. Nigris, *Proceedings of the National Academy of Sciences, March 2005, Vol. 102, pages 4896-4901.*

Erectile dysfunction (ED) in men means damage has occurred in the small, peripheral arteries of the genitals, and thus, ED is a critical warning signal that warrants rejuvenating the arteries with chelation and hormone therapies, especially bio-identical testosterone combined with oxytocin. Other damage includes withering brain neurons that refuse to replicate during aging. Consuming Lithium *prophylactically* (120 mg/d for one month only) increases grey matter by allowing some replication.

Fourthly, none of the above will reliably work if one refuses to exercise for at least a half hour daily. Preferably, you should engage in several hours of walking exercise, a practice common everywhere in the industrial world except in the US. And by exercise, I exclude *heavy aerobics* that burn pounds of oxygen and create cascades of damaging free radicals. Your health, slowed aging, and future depend upon *minimizing free radicals and accompanying inflammation.* I would not appear biologically young at my present age of more than six decades without my one pill/one meal regimen of free-radical scavenger protection used since 1979. I use only 250 mg of l-methionine, l-glutathione, BHT, or l-acetyl cysteine with every meal.

All of these steps can only be achieved with regular *measurement* employing 24 hour urine tests and occasional blood and saliva tests. Regular measurement allows accurate assessment and enhancement of your hormones. Using urine testing, measurement remains critical if one hopes to slow aging and its accompanying indignities.

Lastly, if you expect to live a long and healthy life, you will need to maintain an active sex life combined with a very positive attitude. Everyone has their own methods and choices for these worthy goals, but mine start with the supplementation of bio-identical testosterone, a little thyroid hormone, and some oxytocin (5 units sublingually daily). This sets the body and brain on the path of enhanced libido and friendly, engaging attitudes. Oxytocin makes you bond with your partner and love ones. Without these key hormones many may expect unwanted PMS or IMS (irritable male syndrome); in other words, grumpiness during one's senior years. The hormone oxytocin also increases sexual response and frequency of orgasms in women. Alternatively, for enhanced orgasms women might use a vaginal cream which contains Viagra®, cinnamon oil, and the amino acid, l-arginine. 15 mg daily of the hormone DHEA further enhances libido.

Humor and joy are of critical importance to longevity. The 104 year-old New York philanthropist, Mary Astor always had the right attitude relative to British Queen Victoria. Ms. Astor once said "We are all amused; we are all very amused". And you should be too!

Regarding ongoing illnesses, you should avoid therapies that offer only temporary fixes for your symptoms. Instead, you need to address the ***underlying causes*** of those symptoms with the best that anti-aging medicine offers, namely special nutrients, chelation, free-radical scavengers, eating and exercising right, anti-cross linkers, and the other suggestions that I offer in this book.

Temporary versus Permanent Solutions
I now realize that some major diseases can be largely solved even today if current medical literature were read and applied.

I recently heard a speech by a Hollywood celebrity who made a statement of great impact. Sadly, she explained that all her friends around 60 years of age had at least one medical problem for which orthodox medicine could only offer temporary or marginal solutions.

I know this feeling. All of my friends who ignored anti-aging medicine have found themselves in the same boat. Everyone is destined to die, but those who ignore anti-aging medicine have doomed themselves to suffer needlessly in the decades leading up to the inevitable. You decide. I choose an amusing, friendly, happy life that avoids doom.

In conclusion, consider people who have managed to live 90 or 100 years in relative good health. Ask yourself why. I have my own explanation. These seniors have lacked my anti-aging interventions, but they have lived long lives due to *good health habits and adequate* *endogenous hormones that have sustained them to the century mark.* Their habits and natural endowments you can adapt yourself by joining my carousel of healthy multiple therapies.

Anti-aging medicine resides in a place that is constantly evolving and becoming mainstream. It speaks for the hope that our lives can become richer and more sustaining through uncompromising medical intelligence. This book attempts to soar the panoramic altitudes of that intelligence and assemble the best available therapies by applying a multidisciplinary approach. My approach looms large over the horizon of good health and slowed aging.

This book began with a statement that all major diseases will be curable by the year 2026. After careful examination of the scientific literature, I have changed my mind. I now realize that *some* major diseases can be largely solved *even today* if current medical literature were read and applied. Much of medical practice today is out of touch with the current scientific literature and can be at least 10 to 15 years out of date. For example, 58% of all breast and uterine cancer can be prevented by consuming prophylactically 0.1 mg Arimidix® three times weekly or the topical herb chrysin (50 mg). These doses limit the horrendous carcinogen, *16 alpha hydroxyestrone.* Secondly, 26 different forms of cancer can be avoided by consuming high dose Vitamin D3.

A Parting Example
Genuine testosterone and not its synthetic derivatives will cure your lack of libido, enhance your mood, and reverse many cardiovascular problems.

I would like to present a parting example of the importance of my four hormone horsemen. I wish to demonstrate their importance to longevity and good health during one's senior years. Consider testosterone (T). During WWI, a Danish physician attached the testicles of a dead soldier to a man suffering from gangrene. The extra testicles generated enough T to cure the gangrene and saved his appendages from amputation. The patient's blood became *oxygenated* from near zero to 100% when extra T was introduced. In later years in Denmark, Dr. Jens Møller and colleagues applied injectable T and saved many patients from gangrene and a *host of other cardiovascular diseases* during a forty year period. Anti-aging physicians have rediscovered this treatment by applying bio-identical T in the form of a cream or gel 50 to 100 mg daily in men and one twelfth this dose in women. Genuine testosterone and not its synthetic derivatives will cure your lack of libido, enhance your mood, and reverse many cardiovascular problems. Add a cup daily of pomegranate juice and 50,000 units weekly of Vitamin D3 and experience lower blood pressure by about 12 mm mercury. This is my Lippman Promise.

Life should be an exciting, amazing adventure with new joys and experiences every waking day and with every turn in the road. Find yourself an anti-aging physician through a compounding-pharmacy referral and join the revolution.

Golden keys to longevity # 14

- *For most people the only way to extend their lives to 90, 100, or beyond is to **measure and balance** their hormones using 24 hour urine tests. These tests determine no less than 29 hormones and their metabolites. Special vitamins such as B12, D3, and hormones such as testosterone, progesterone, oxytocin, and thyroid remain critical to health and longevity. Deadly carcinogens can be prevented by applying the **current** medical literature.*

Recommendations

- No recommendations of hormone therapy can be made unless patients are first tested, especially with 24 hour urine tests.

Chapter 15
Resources

Sourcing Supplements and Physicians

1. Sourcing board-certified or knowledgeable anti-aging physician contact: 1) the best way: contact your local compounding pharmacist and ask them for physician referrals in your area of the US. 2) second best: log onto www.worldhealth.net/event/php or telephone 561-997-0112 and ask for two charming ladies (Danielle Goldstein or Sandra Lopez) at American Academy of Anti-Aging Medicine, 301 Yamato Road Ste. 2160, Boca Raton, FL 33431

2. Most ingredients can be purchased from any full-service health food store. Otherwise, I can enthusiastically recommend the following:

3. www.vrp.com (complete selection of the best anti-aging nutritional products in the USA).

4. www.antiaging-motivate.com (preferred source of exotic anti-aging products not easily available in the US).

5. www.swansonvitamins.com (inexpensive vitamins and nutrients).

6. Costco (inexpensive vitamins).

7. www.meridianvalleylab.com (favorite lab for 24 hour urine testing).

8. www.womensinternational.com (highly respected supplier of bio-identical hormones)
9. www.keynutritionrx.com (bio-identical hormones and especially *aldosterone*).
10. www.youngagainproducts.com (various bio-identical creams).
11. www.betterhealthinternational.com (bio-identical progesterone creams).
12. www.allstarhealth.com (chromium polynicotinate source).
13. University Compounding Pharmacy, 1875 Third Ave., San Diego, CA 92101, tel. 800-985-8065, full service bio-identical hormones, especially *oxytocin*.
14. Century Square Pharmacy, 1188 Bishop St. #2303, Honolulu, HI (full service bio-identical hormones).
15. Marukai Store, Ward Warehouse, Honolulu, HI (favorite Japanese-American market for healthy Japanese and American foods (ask for Denise in the supplements section).
16. Teshima's Restaurant, 79-7251 Mamalahoa Hwy., Kealakekua, HI (my favorite Japanese-American Restaurant for truly healthy food, especially traditional Japanese breakfast. The owner, Mrs. Teshima is 101 years old, and since 1929 she has worked there. Her longevity attests to the superb quality of her traditional Japanese food.)

Section 4

Appendix: Medical References

Antioxidants and Free Radical Scavengers

J. of Gerontology, 1965, Harman, D, 20, pp. 151-153.
J. of the Am. Geriatrics Soc., 1969, Harman, D, 17, pp. 721-735.
J. of Gerontology, 1980, Leibovitz, B. & Siegal, BV, 35, pp. 45-56.
Photochemistry & Photobiology, 1978, Pryor, WA, 28, pp. 787-801.
J. of Gerontology, 1973, Tappel, AL, 28, pp. 415-424.
Proc. Natl. Acad. Sci. USA, 1981, Harman, D, 73, pp. 7124-7128.
Forskning och Framsteg, 1981, Uhlén, M. & Lippman, R.D, 1, pp. 24-27.

J. of Gerontology, 1981, Vol. 36, No. 5, pp. 550-557. Lippman, R.D. The Prolongation of Life: A Comparison of Antioxidants and Geroprotectors versus Superoxide in Human Mitochondria.

Mechanisms of Ageing and Development, 1981, Vol. 17, pp. 283-287.
Lippman, RD, et. al., Application of Chemiluminescent Probes in Investigating Lysosomal Sensitivity to Superoxide versus Suspected Radical Scavengers.

Review of Biological Research in Aging, Alan R. Liss, Inc., NY, NY, 1983, Vol. 1, pp. 315-342.
Lippman, RD, Lipid Peroxidation and Metabolism in Aging: A Biological, Chemical, and Medical Approach.

Oxygen Radicals in Chemistry and Biology, 1984, Walter de Gruyter & Co., Berlin, pp.736-740.
Lippman, RD, Measurement of Lipid Hydroperoxides and Collagen Elasticity Directly *in vivo* In Mice and Man.

US Patent Nr. 4695590, 1987, Lippman, RD, Method for Retarding Human Aging.

Cross-Linking or Glycation

Chem. Industries, 1941, Björksten, J, 48, pp. 746-751.
J. Am. Geriatrics Soc., 1958, Björksten, J, 6, pp. 740-747.

J. Am. Geriatrics Soc, 1960, Björksten, J. & Andrews, F, 8, pp. 632-637.
Comprehensive Therapy, 1978, Björksten, J, 4, pp. 44-52.
Rejuvenation, 1980, Carpenter, D, 7, pp. 31-49.
New England J. of Medicine, 1988, 318, pp. 1315-1321.
Annals of Med, 1996, 28, pp. 419-426.
Exp. Eye Research, 1996, 62, pp. 505-510.
Stroke, 1996, 27, pp. 1393-1398.
Biochem. Biophy. Res. Comm, 1999, 257, pp. 251-258.
Diabetalogia, 2001, 44(1), pp. 108-114.
Circulation, 2001 Sept, 25, 104(13), pp. 1464-1470.
Diabetes, 2002, 51, pp. 2826-2832.
Arch. Biochem. Biophys, 2003, 419, pp. 41-49.

Bio-identical Hormone Replacement

Biomedicina, 2000 Jan; Vol. 3 (1), pp.6-7.
Maturitas, 1999 Aug;16 32(3), pp. 147-153.

Testosterone

International Journal of Obesity and Metabolic Disorders, 1992 Dec; 16(12), pp. 991-997.
Medical Crossfire, 2001 Jan; Vol.3 No.1, pp. 17, 18, 47-50.
Diabetes Care 2003 June; Vol. 36, No.6, pp. 20-30.
Archives of Family Medicine, 1999, Vol.8, pp. 252-263.
RRJ Cancer 1999 June; 80(7), pp. 930-934.
Cancer 1999, July 15;88(2), pp. 312-315.
New England Journal of Medicine 2004; 350, pp. 482-492.
New England Journal of Medicine, 2000; 343, pp. 682-688.
Diabetes Metab. 1995, Vol. 21, pp. 156-161.
J. Natl. Med. Assoc. Sept, 2000; 92(9), pp. 445-449.
Am. J. of Epidemiology, 2002; 155, pp. 437-445.
Consultant, 1999 August, pp. 2006-2007.
JAMA, May 2004; Vol. 283(20), pp. 2463-2464.
Diabetes Care, 2003; Vol. 26, No. 6, pp. 1869-1876.
Neurology, 2005, Mar. 8; 64-65, pp. 866-871.
Atherosclerosis, 1996, Mar; 121(1); pp. 35-43.

Female Patient, 2004, Nov; Vol. 29, pp.40-45.

Diabetes Metab. 2004 Feb; 30(1), pp. 29-34.

Obesity Review 2004, Nov; 5(4), pp. 197-216.

Female Patient 2004, Nov. Vol. 29, pp. 40-45.

J. of Reproductive Medicine, 1999; 44(12), pp. 1012-1020.

J. of Urology, 2003, 170, pp. 2348-2351.

New England J Med, 2004; 350, pp. 482-492.

Mayo Clin Proc, 2002, Jan;75, pp. 583-587.

Brit. J. Urology, 1990 Mar; 77(3), pp. 437-443.

Obestiy Reps, 1995, 3, pp. 6098-6125.

J. of Clinical Endocrin. Metabolism, 2008, Vol. 93, No. 1, pp. 68-75
and pp. 139-146.

Testosterone Treatment of Cardiovascular Diseases, 1984, Jens
Møller & H. Einfeldt, Springer-Verlag, Germany.

*Cholesterol: Interactions with Testosterone and Cortisol in
Cardiovascular Diseases*, 1987, Jens Møller, Springer-Verlag,
Germany.

Progesterone

Female Patient, 2001 Oct, pp. 19-21

Infertility & Reproductive Medicine Clinics of North America, 1995
Oct, Vol. 6(4), pp. 653-673.

Am. Family Physicians, 2000, 62, pp. 1339-1346.

Am. J. Obstetric Gynecology, 1999 Jan., 180, pp. 42-48.

Nat. Academy Science USA, 2003 Sept.2, 100(8), pp. 10506-10511.

Obstetrics Gynecology, 1989, 73, pp. 606.

Am. J. Obstetrics Gynecology, 1999 Jan, 180, pp. 42-48.

Circulation, 1999 Dec, 100, pp. 2319-2325.

Cortland Forum, 2000 July, pp. 170-174.

Infertility and Reproductive Clinics of North Am, 1995 Oct, 6(4), pp.
653-667.

JAMA, 2000, 203, pp. 485-91.

Family Practice News, 2004 March, 15, pp. 1-3.

Proturitor, 2003 Dec, 46(1), pp. 555-558.

Clinical Therapy, 1999 Jan, 21(1), pp. 41-60.

J. of Women's Health Gender Based Med, 2000 May, 9(4), pp. 381-
387.

Maturitas, 2003 Dec, 46(1), pp. 555-558.

Am. Family Physician, 2000, 62, pp. 1939-1946.

Obstetrics Gynecology, 1989, 73, pp. 606-611.

Climacteric, 2002 Sept, 5(3), pp. 229-235.

J. Women's Health Gender Based Med, 2000 May, 9(4), pp. 381-387.

J. Am. College of Cardiology, 2000 Dec, 36(9), pp. 2154-2159.

Breast Cancer Res. Treat, 2007 Feb, pp. 160-175.

Am. Family Physician, 2000, 62, pp. 1839-1846.

Fertility Sterility, 1998, 69, pp. 963-969.

Japan J. of Cancer Research, 1985 June, 76, pp. 699-704.

Infertility and Reproductive Med. Clinics of North Am, 1995 Oct, 6(4), pp. 653-670.

J. Nat. Cancer Institute, 2000, 92(4), pp. 328-332.

Climateric, 2003 Sept, 6, pp. 221-227.

Estrogen

Circulation, 2001, 104, pp. 499-503.

Infertility and Reproductive Med. Clinics of North Am, 1995 Oct, Vol.6(4), pp. 653-675.

JAMA, 2004, 291(24), pp. 2947-2958.

Hospital Practice, 1999 Aug, pp. 295-305.

Fam. Practice News, 2005 March, pp. 58-59.

Obstet. Gynecology, 1996 Jan, 87(1), pp. 6-12.

Female Patient, 2004 Oct, Vol. 29, pp. 40-46.

Biomedica, 2000 Jan, Vol. 3(1), pp. 6-9.

Obstetrics Gynecology, 1989 April, 73, pp. 606-611.

Obstetrics Gynecology, 1996 Jan, 87(1), pp. 6-12.

Consultant, 2001 July, Vol. 71, pp. 1085-1086.

Circulation, 1998 Sept, 98(12), pp. 1158-1163.

Nat. Academy of Science USA, 1997, 94, pp. 6612-6617.

Female Patient, 2001 April, 26. pp. 18-24.

JAMA, 2002 Aug, Vol. 288, No.7, pp. 880-887.

Female Patient, 2004 Oct, Vol. 29, pp. 35-41.

J. Gen. Internal Med, 2004, 19(7), pp. 791-804.

Family Practice News, 2003 June, Vol. 33(11), pp. 1-2.

Nat. Academy of Science USA, 1997, 94, pp. 6612-6617.

Female Patient, 2001 April, 26, pp. 18-24.

JAMA, 2002 August, Vol. 288, No. 7, pp. 880-887.

Female Patient, 2004 Oct, Vol. 29, pp. 35-41.

J. Gen. Internal Med, 2004, 19(7), pp. 791-804.

Family Practice News, 2003 June, Vol. 33(11), pp. 1-2.

JAMA, 2002 August, Vol. 288, pp. 2123-2129.

Obesity Review, 2004 Nov, 5(4), pp. 197-216.

Postgraduate Med., 2000 Sept, 108(3), pp. 147-150.

New England J. of Medicine, 2000, 343(8), pp. 572-574.

Clinical Genetics, 1998 May, 6(5), pp. 15-19.

Breast Cancer Research Treat, 2007, 101, pp. 125-134.

Fertility Sterility, 2005 Dec, 84(6), pp. 1589-1601.

Female Patient, 2004 Oct, Vol. 29, pp. 40-46.

Family Practice News, 2003 Oct, pp. 1-2.

Female Patient, 2001 April, 26, pp. 18-24.

New England J. of Medicine, 2000, 343(8), pp. 572-574.

Clinical Genetics, 1998 Med, 6(5), pp. 15-19.

Thyroid

Med. Hypothesis, 2003 Aug, 21(2), pp. 182-189.

J. Clinical Endocrin. Metabolism, 2005 May, 90(5), pp. 2666-2674.

Cortland Forum, 2001 July, pp. 85-90.

British Med. J., 2003 Feb, Vol. 326, pp. 325-326.

Normal Metabolic Research, 1995 Nov, 27(11), pp. 503-507.

British Med. J, 2003 Feb, Vol. 326, pp. 295-296.

New England J. of Medicine, 1999 Feb, pp. 424-429.

Annals of Internal Med, 2000, 132, pp. 270-278.

CVR & R, 2002, 23, pp. 20-26.

JAMA, 2004 Dec, Vol. 292(2c), pp. 500-504.

Consultant, 2000 Dec, pp. 2397-2399.

Lancet, 1992 Jul, 4, 340(8810), pp. 9-13.

J. of Gerontology, 1999, Vol. 54, pp. 109-115.

J. of Clinical Endocrine Metabolism, 2005 May, 90(5), pp. 2666-2674.

Cortland Forum, 2001 July, pp. 85-89.

Preventive Cardiology, 2001, 4, pp. 179-182.

Melatonin

Med. Hypothesis, 1997 June, 49(6), pp. 523-535.
Patient Care, 2000 June, pp. 34-38.
Archives of Internal Med, 1999 Nov. 159, pp. 2456-2460.
J. Pineal Research, 1999 Aug, 23(i), pp. 15-19.
Neurology, 2004 Aug, pp. 246-250.

Cancer

J. of Steroid Biochem. Mol. Biology, 2005 May, Pub Med.
J. of Obstet. Gynecology, 2004 Jan, 23(1), pp. 49-60.
Menopause, 2003 Jul-Aug, 10(4), pp. 269-270 & 292-298.
Am. J. Physiol. Endocrine Metabolism, 2005 Dec, Pub Med.
FEBS LETT, 2005 Oct, 579(25), pp. 5535-5541.
Female Patient, 2001 Dec, pp. 3-10.
Breast Cancer Research Treat, 2007, pp. 125-134.
J. Clin. Epidemiol, 2004 Aug, 57(8), pp. 766-772.
Cancer, 2003, 97, pp.1387-1392.
JAMA, 1966, 196(13), pp. 1128-1136.
Curr. Opin. Oncol, 2005 Sep, 17(5) pp. 493-499.
Menopause, 2004 Sept-Oct, 11(5), pp. 531-535.
British J. of Cancer, 1996, 73, pp. 1552-1555.
New England J. of Medicine, 2004, Vol. 351, No. 26, pp. 2773-2774.

2-Methoxy Estradiol Versus Cancer

Epidemology, 2000 Nov. 11(6), pp. 635-640.
J. Natl. Cancer Inst, 1999 June, 19(12), pp. 1067-1072.
Bone, 2004 Sept, 35(3), pp. 682-688.
Endocrinol. Metab, 2005 April, 90(4), pp. 2035-2041.
J. Rheumatol, 2004 Mar, 31(3), pp. 489-494.
Environ. Health Perspect, 1995 Oct, 103 (suppl. 7), pp. 147-150.

Tinley TL, Leal RM, Randall-Hlubek DA, et al. "Novel 2-methoxyestradiol analogues with antitumor activity." *Cancer Research 2003*; 63: 1,538-1,549.

Pribluda VS, Gubish ER Jr., Lavallee TM, et al. "2-methoxyestradiol: an endogenous antiangiogenic and antiproliferative drug candidate." *Cancer Metastasis Rev 2000*; 19(1-2): 173-179.

Golebiewska J, Rozwadowski P, Spodnik JH, et al. "Dual effect of 2-methoxyestradiol on cell cycle events in human osteosarcoma 143 B cells." *Acta Biochemica Polonica 2002*; 49(1): 59-65.

Drissa A, Bennani H, Giton F, et al. "Tocopherols and saponins derived from Argania spinosa exert an antiproliferative effect on human prostate cancer." *Cancer Invest 2006*; 24(6): 588-592.

Mueck AO, Seeger H, Huober J. "Chemotherapy of breast cancer-additive anticancerogenic effects by 2-methoxyestradiol?" *Life Sci 2004*; 75(10): 1,205-1,210.

Gomez LA, de Las Pozas A, Reiner T, et al. "Increased expression of cyclin B1 sensitizes prostate cancer cells to apoptosis induced by chemotherapy." *Mol Cancer Ther 2007*;6(5): 1,534-1,543.

Schumacher G, Hoffmann J, Cramer T, et al. "Antineoplastic activity of 2-methoxyestradiol in human pancreatic and gastric cancer cells with different multidrug-resistant phenotypes." *J Gastroenterol Hepatol 2007*; 22(9): 1,469-1,473

Mueck AO, Seeger H, Wallwiener D, Huober J. "Is the combination with 2-methoxyestradiol able to reduce the dosages of chemotherapeutics in the treatment of human ovarian cancer? Preliminary in vitro investigations." *Eur J Gynaecol Oncol 2004*; 25(6): 699-701.

Golebiewska J, Rozwadowski P, Spodnik JH, et al. "Dual effect of 2-methoxyestradiol on cell cycle events in human osteosarcoma 143 B cells." *Acta Biochemica Polonica 2002*; 49(1): 59-65.

Shogren KL, Turner RT, Yaszemski J, Maran A. "Double-stranded RNA-dependent protein kinase is involved in 2-methoxyestradiol-mediated cell death of osteosarcoma cells." *J Bone Miner Res 2007*: 22(1): 29-36.

She MR, Li JG, Guo KY, et al. "Requirement of reactive oxygen species generation in apoptosis of leukemia cells induced by 2-methoxyestradiol." *Acta Pharmacologica Sinica 2007*; 28(7): 1,037-1,044.

Fong YC, Yang WH, Hsu SF, et al. "2-methoxyestradiol induces apoptosis and cell cycle arrest in human chondrosarcoma cells." *J Orthop Res 2007*; 25(8): 1,106-1,114.

Miller KD, Haney LG, Pribluda VS, Sledge VW. "A phase I safety, pharmacokinetic and pharmacodynamic study of 2-methoxyestradiol (2ME2) in patients with refractory metastatic breast cancer." *Proceedings of the American Society of Clinical Oncology 2001*; 170: 20-43a.

Davoodpour P, Landstrom M, Welsh M. "Reduced tumor growth in vivo and increased c-Abl activity in PC3 prostate cancer cells overexpressing the Shb adapter protein." *BMC Cancer 2007*; 7: 161.

Ho A, Kim YE, Lee H, et al. "SAR studies of 2-methoxyestradiol and development of its analogs as probes of anti-tumor mechanisms." *Bioorg Med Chem Lett 2006*; 16(13): 3,383-3,387.

Tinley TL, Leal RM, Randall-Hlubek DA, et al. "Novel 2-methoxyestradiol analogues with antitumor activity." *Cancer Research 2003*; 63: 1,538-1,549. 17 "Drug found effective in treating, preventing breast cancer," *Science Daily* (www.sciencedaily.com), 11/4/07.

Cicek M, Iwaniec UT, Goblirsch MJ, et al. "2-methoxyestradiol suppresses osteolytic breast cancer tumor progression in vivo." *Cancer Res 2007*; 67(21): 10,106-10,111.

19 Miller KD, Haney LG, Pribluda VS, Sledge VW. "A phase I safety, pharmacokinetic and pharmacodynamic study of 2-methoxyestradiol (2ME2) in patients with refractory metastatic breast cancer." *Proceedings of the American Society of Clinical Oncology 2001*; 170: 20-43a.

Miller KD, Haney LG, Pribluda VS, et al. "A phase I study of 2-methoxyestradiol (2ME2) plus docetaxel in patients with metastatic breast cancer." *Proceedings of the American Society of Clinical Oncology 2002*; 21: 111a.

Dahut W, Lakhani NJ, Gulley JL, et al. "Phase I clinical trial of oral 2-methoxyestradiol, an antiangiogenic and apoptotic agent, in patients with solid tumors." *Cancer Biology & Therapy 2006*; 5(1): 22-27.

Sweeney C, Liu G, Yiannoutsos C, et al. "A phase II multicenter, randomized, double-blind, safety trial assessing the pharmacokinetics, pharmacodynamics, and efficacy of oral 2-methoxyestradiol capsules in hormone-refractory prostate cancer." *Clinical Cancer Research 2005*; 11: 6,625-6,633.

Salama SA, et al. "Estrogen metabolite 2-Methoxyestradiol induces apoptosis and inhibits cell proliferation and collagen production in rat and human leiomyoma cells: a potential medicinal treatment for uterine fibroids." *J Soc Gynecol Invest 2006*; 13: 542-550.

Estriol

JAMA, 1966, 196(13), pp. 1128-1136.
Mol. Endocrinol, 1997 Nov, 11(12), pp. 1868-18-78.
Lancet, 1973 Mar, 1(7802), pp. 546-547.

DHEA (dihydro-epiandrosterone)

JAMA, 2004, 292, pp. 2243-2248.
J. Clin. Endocrine Metabolism, 1999 June, 84(6), pp. 2008-2012.
J. Rheumatology, 1988, 25(2), pp. 285-289.

Biological Psychiatry, 1997, 41(3) pp. 311-318.
Annals N.Y. Academy of Science, 1995 Dec, 774, pp. 271-280.
New England J. of Medicine, 1986 Dec, 315(24), pp. 1519-1524.
J. of Clinical Invest, 1988, 82(2), pp. 712-720.
J. of Clinical Endrocrin. Metab., 1997 June, 78(6), pp. 1360-1367.
J. of Clinical Endrocrin. Metab, 1997 Oct, 82(10), pp. 3498-3505.
Am. J. Pyschiatry, 1999, 150, pp. 646-649.
JAMA, 2004 Nov, Vol. 29(18), pp. 2233-2247.
J. Am. Gerontology Soc, 1999 June, 47(6), pp. 685-691.
Am. J. Psychiatry, 1999 April, 156(4), pp. 646-649.
J. Psych, 2000 Dec, 85(12), pp. 4650-4656.
Endocrinology Research, 2000 Nov, 26(4), p. 505.
Critical Care Med., 2001 Feb, 29(2), p. 380.
Clinical Endocrinology, 1998 Oct, 49(4), pp. 421-432.
J. Family Med, 1988 Jan, 60(1), pp. 57-81.
Am. J. Health Syst. Pharm, 57(22), pp. 2048-2056.
Clin. Endomet, 1994 June, 78(6), pp. 1360-1367.

Glandular Extracts

Urol. & Cutan. Review, 1929 Nov, xxxiii, p. 724.
Proc. Staff Meetings of the Mayo Clinic, 1933 Aug 9, viii, p. 481.
Glaucoma and It's Medical Treatment with Cortin, 1937, Emanuel Josephson, Chedney Press, New York City.
Introduction to Cellular Therapy, 1960, Paul Niehans, Pageant Books, New York.
Hypoadrenocorticism, 1980, John Tintera, Adrenal Metabolic Research Society, Troy, N.Y.
Proto-Endocrinology, 1983, J. Needham & G-D Lu, Vol. 5, Part 5, Cambridge Univ. Press, UK.

HGH (human growth hormone):
156,000 PubMed hits on 2-01-08. The most significant:

JAMA, 2000 Aug, 284(7), pp. 879-881.
Gerontology, 2002 Nov-Dec, 48(6), pp. 401-417.
J Clinical Endocrin Metab, 2001 Sep, 86(9), pp. 4139-4146.
J Clinical Endocrin Metab, 2003 Aug, 88(8), pp. 3663-3667.

Treat Endocrin, 2006, 5(3), pp. 159-157.

Front Neuroendocrin, 2000 Oct, 21(4), pp. 330-348.

J of Neuroscience, 2001 Mar, 21(6), pp. 1902-1910.

J Clinical Endocrin Metab, 1999 June, 84(6), pp. 1919-1924.

Growth Horm 1GF Res, 2006 May, p. 9.

Eur J Endocrin, 2000 Nov, 143(5), pp. 585-592.

Ann Intern Med, 1996 Dec, 125(11), pp. 883-890.

J Clinical Endocrin Metab, 2007 Aug, p.14.

J Clinical Endocrin Metab, 2004 Jan, 89(1), pp. 114-120.

Pediatr Nephrol, 2004 Nov 4.

Am Heart J, 2002 Aug, 144(2), pp. 359-364.

Horm Res, 2000 July, 53 Suppl S1, pp. 87-97.

JAMA, 2002 July, Vol. 288, No. 18.

J Clinical Endocrin Metab, 2004 Feb, 89(2), pp. 695-701.

J Clinical Endocrin Metab, 2005 Mar, 90(3), pp. 1466-1474.

CPSIA information can be obtained at www.ICGtesting.com
Printed in the USA
LVOW080735091112

306608LV00002B/1/P